RISK AND ADAPTATION IN A CANCER CLUSTER TOWN

NATURE, SOCIETY, AND CULTURE

Scott Frickel, Series Editor

A sophisticated and wide-ranging sociological literature analyzing nature-society-culture interactions has blossomed in recent decades. This book series provides a platform for showcasing the best of that scholarship: carefully crafted empirical studies of socio-environmental change and the effects such change has on ecosystems, social institutions, historical processes, and cultural practices.

The series aims for topical and theoretical breadth. Anchored in sociological analyses of the environment, Nature, Society, and Culture is home to studies employing a range of disciplinary and interdisciplinary perspectives and investigating the pressing socio-environmental questions of our time—from environmental inequality and risk, to the science and politics of climate change and serial disaster, to the environmental causes and consequences of urbanization and war making, and beyond.

For a list of all the titles in the series, please see the last page of the book.

RISK AND ADAPTATION IN A CANCER CLUSTER TOWN

LAURA HART

RUTGERS UNIVERSITY PRESS
New Brunswick, Camden, and Newark, New Jersey
London and Oxford

Rutgers University Press is a department of Rutgers, The State University of New Jersey, one of the leading public research universities in the nation. By publishing worldwide, it furthers the University's mission of dedication to excellence in teaching, scholarship, research, and clinical care.

Library of Congress Cataloging-in-Publication Data

Names: Hart, Laura (Laura B.), author.
Title: Risk and adaptation in a cancer cluster town / Laura Hart.
Description: New Brunswick, New Jersey : Rutgers University Press, [2023] |
    Includes bibliographical references and index.
Identifiers: LCCN 2022040556 | ISBN 9781978823532 (paperback) |
    ISBN 9781978823549 (hardback) | ISBN 9781978823556 (epub) |
    ISBN 9781978823570 (pdf)
Subjects: LCSH: Belonging (Social psychology) | Communities. | Equality. |
    Environmental risk assessment. | Chemical industry—Waste disposal—
    Environmental aspects.
Classification: LCC HM1033 .H386 2023 | DDC 302—dc23/eng/20220913
LC record available at https://lccn.loc.gov/2022040556

A British Cataloging-in-Publication record for this book is available from the British Library.

References to internet websites (URLs) were accurate at the time of writing. Neither the author nor Rutgers University Press is responsible for URLs that may have expired or changed since the manuscript was prepared.

♾ The paper used in this publication meets the requirements of the American National Standard for Information Sciences—Permanence of Paper for Printed Library Materials, ANSI Z39.48-1992.

rutgersuniversitypress.org

This book is dedicated to the children and families at the center of this story.

CONTENTS

PREFACE AND ACKNOWLEDGMENTS

Winesburg, Ohio is a 1919 collection of short stories by Sherwood Anderson. The fictional town of Winesburg is based on the writer's memories of his own town, Clyde, Ohio—the town that is also the focus of this book. The prevailing mood in *Winesburg, Ohio* is one of misunderstanding and loneliness, restlessness, dissatisfaction, and disillusionment. There is no real sense of community in this fictional town; most of the characters in Winesburg are portrayed in a moment of crisis, and no one is able to achieve meaningful understanding of another person. As observed by journalist Kristina Smith's *Ohio Magazine* article "'Winesburg, Ohio' at 100," it's not surprising that residents of Clyde were not always proud of Anderson's scandalous portrayal of the town.[1] Early in my fieldwork I wondered if there was something about the town that still fostered the absence of community that Anderson so accurately captures. This assumption was contradicted by resident after resident who ecstatically told me that Clyde was the best community in which to live. Nonetheless, I see an interplay between structural forces and something more intimate—a passivity that is not easy to describe considering the health crisis faced by the community. It is characterized by fear of the loss of security and fear of the unknown—both material and social. In some manifestations, it is characterized by a lack of loyalty that makes for shifty alliances. In others, it appears as loneliness so profound that their connection to others is compromised altogether. This book is an attempt, in the complex field of qualitative data, to edge closer to an understanding of how life politics are negotiated.

About 1,000 suspected cancer clusters are annually reported to state health departments. When I ask my students about disease clusters, they often share stories about perceived clusters of illness in or near their hometowns. My hometown is no exception. My brother remembers the summer the cornfield was sprayed next to our house and the "whole neighborhood talking about their throats." Another relative has a father with MS, who grew up on a road where three other people were diagnosed with the same disease. My mother, who taught art at a public high school, had more than one student from the same neighborhood present with a rare form of bone cancer. My father was diagnosed with cancer, and we suspected that it was linked to Agent Orange exposure when he was stationed in the DMZ in Korea during the Vietnam War. Years later, the federal government would recognize this connection, but my questions about the relationship between toxins and disease and adaptation to illness grew. These experiences reinforced my belief that peripheral issues related to disease are profound. The social, behavioral, economic, cultural, and environmental variations in health and disease are as important as biomedical ones.

This book was born of the inspiration of many people and has been shaped by all those willing to listen and make suggestions. Its earliest genesis was in the lively intellectual and activist-oriented department of Sociology at Humboldt State University. I would not be who I am had I not had the privilege of working with Mary Virnoche and Jennifer Eichstedt, who taught me how to ask critical questions and to prioritize dialogue and community, and Sing Chew, who deepened my understanding of social theory. In Arcata, California, the women whom I interviewed for my master's thesis about their experiences with cancer also pushed me to think about new questions about how institutions infiltrate into our experiences and the meanings we attach to them.

This book began as a dissertation in the University of Illinois Urbana-Champaign's (UIUC) Sociology department, where it benefited from the confluence of smart people. I particularly thank my dissertation advisor, Moon-Kie Jung, who provided this project with wise guidance and encouraged me to think about this project as a book. I also thank readers Assata Zerai, Lisa Cacho, and Norman Denzin, who each, in their own ways, pushed me to sharpen my analysis of power and how it intersects with social justice. I also extend my appreciation to Maryalice Wu, Dawn Owens, and Kathleen Santa Ana at UIUC for training me to be analytically careful and for mentoring me through the lifecycle of many research projects.

The research of this book was aided by the American Sociological Foundation (ASA) Fund for the Advancement of the Discipline (FAD) grant, as well as a summer research stipend from Missouri State University. I would like to especially acknowledge my first-rate research assistant, Jessica Powell; I would likely still be swimming in the transdisciplinary literature if it weren't for her many organized and comprehensive literature reviews. I also thank Callyn Broyles for her help with interview transcription.

For permission to reproduce copyright materials, I thank the Charles E. Burchfield Foundation, the Hagley Museum & Library, and Gene Smith at the Clyde Heritage League. I thank cartographer Mike Siegel in the Geography Department at Rutgers University for creating a map for me.

While working on the book, I was lucky to have the support and feedback of friends and colleagues. I presented parts of this research to a number of audiences, all of whom helped it immeasurably. I thank Kari Norgaard for her encouragement for this project during our panel on Emotional Politics of Environmental Threats at the ASA in Philadelphia in 2018. Both her scholarship in this area and her collectivist kindness have left an impression on me.

I want to thank my editor, Peter Mickulas, for his guidance and enthusiasm about this project. I also thank Peter for choosing my excellent reviewers. My anonymous reviewer and my non-anonymous reviewer, Peter Little, offered detailed, incisive critiques that helped immeasurably. I want to also thank Candida Hadley, whose developmental editing insights, recommendations, and encouragement helped me make this a much better book. And thanks for an extremely careful job to production editor Brian Ostrander at Westchester Publishing Services and copy editor Ellen Lohman.

I am also very lucky to have strong writers in my family and in my circle of nonacademic friends. I extend my deepest appreciation to my mother, Judy Atkins, for spending countless hours reading every chapter, and for also providing childcare so that I could move my project toward completion. I also wish to thank my father, Alex Atkins, my brother Jesse Atkins, and my sister-in-law Arianna Atkins for their encouragement. I acknowledge my late grandmother, Tillie Atkins— also a sociologist by training. The photo of her in my office often reminded me that I, too, could overcome obstacles. To Angie Carvalho, I owe a special thanks for her generous readings and proofreading and for her friendship.

For the eight years that it took me to complete this project—during which I had two children—my husband, Nathan Hart, lived with my uncertainties. I thank Nathan for carrying the childcare responsibilities—sometimes exclusively—so I could write on weekends. I also thank him for protecting his own playful spirit, and for sharing it with our family, especially at times when I felt overwhelmed. I thank my son and daughter, Jacob and Ava Hart, for their own inherent joyfulness and for providing the meaning and motivation for everything I do.

Finally, in Clyde, I was met with exceptional help. I want to thank the kind family who rented a room to me during the bulk of my data collection. I am grateful to all the individuals whose personal stories and experiences helped me write this book. I am indebted to them for allowing me to narrate their experiences and share their critique, and for being willing to be so candid with me about their experiences of loss.

RISK AND ADAPTATION IN A CANCER CLUSTER TOWN

INTRODUCTION
The Town of Whirlpool

M CPHERSON HIGHWAY RUNS east to west through the town of Clyde, Ohio. It is not Main Street, which runs the opposite direction, but is perhaps a more modernized version of Main Street that now serves as the focal point for retailing and socializing. Both independent and corporately owned businesses stand along McPherson Highway, and, like in many small towns across America, offer services that people need and keep residents local. Clyde is also home to a Whirlpool Corporation plant that manufactures household appliances in a large industrial complex and is the community's largest employer.

Upon approaching Ohio towns like Clyde, one passes fields of soybeans and corn and occasional herds of dairy cattle. Like much of central and northwest Ohio, land surrounding the area of Clyde and the adjacent portions of Green Creek Township in eastern Sandusky County is primarily agricultural. These largely rural areas are situated on a broad, mostly level, glacial lake plain approximately fifteen miles south of Lake Erie. Yet, attentive passersby can now also catch a glimpse of billboards advertising the services of cancer centers, randomly placed indicators of portentous significance at odds with the picturesque scenery. Intrusions such as this now exist within many of these rustic settings and can be seen in the town of Clyde where a Cleveland Clinic Cancer Center is situated across from the Whirlpool factory. Such imagery has now been absorbed into the contemporary landscape.

Residents in present-day Clyde have a long history of family ties to the town. It is an "Everybody knows everybody" type of place. People will describe the many selling points of small-town living—Clyde provides "safety," a peaceful lifestyle, and beautiful nature and is a place where one would want to raise children. Many have fond memories of growing up in the old-fashioned, small-town atmosphere and will share stories about swimming, fishing, mushroom hunting, and duck hunting. While each has memories unique to their experience, there is a commonality about them that evokes nostalgia for a simple way of living.

In spite of appearances, though, Clyde was classified as a cancer cluster in 2009 after the Ohio Department of Health determined that the number of childhood cancers was statistically significantly higher than what would be expected in the area, most likely the result of exposure to environmental toxins. The Centers for Disease Control and Prevention defines disease clusters as an unusual aggregation, real or perceived, of health events that are grouped together in time and space and that are reported to a health agency. Between 1996 and 2010, thirty-five children were diagnosed with or died from cancer in eastern Sandusky County, with several cases presenting since then. Many adults have been diagnosed with unusual cancers as well, although this anomaly is not reflected in the official health assessment conducted in the area.

My entry into the study of Clyde coincided with the filing of a lawsuit by a small number of impacted residents against Whirlpool Corporation after the Environmental Protection Agency (EPA) discovery in 2012 of a toxic dump site composed of polychlorinated biphenyl (PCB) sludge measuring above one part per million and nine feet deep beneath the basketball and tennis courts in Whirlpool Park. This contaminant was also suspected of seeping into the park's swimming pool. Although previously denying responsibility for its being buried in the park, the company did not contest that contaminants were placed there while they owned the property. PCBs are considered carcinogenic and were banned in 1979 because of their links to endocrine disruption and neurotoxicity. Contrary to what many might expect, the lawsuit against the company became more controversial in the town than the discovery of the PCB sludge. I drove to Clyde to attend a public meeting held by the team of lawyers and scientists hired by the families to conduct independent environmental tests.

LITTLE OLD CLYDE

A locally owned diner sat along McPherson Highway and stood out among the decline of other businesses on Main Street. On the morning after the meeting, I stopped at Gary's Diner to organize my research notes before beginning my two-hour drive home. The diner appeared to be converted from a mobile trailer and had elements of a 1950s retro decorative style, including a long sit-down counter with direct service of American staples. It had a very small-town atmosphere and, although there were fewer than ten patrons inside, most of whom were older white men, the atmosphere felt full of the type of civic energy that is characteristic of small-town diners. Almost immediately upon my finding a booth, a man introduced himself to me as the owner and a member of the city council. He enthusiastically offered me his contact information for an interview and took a few of my project flyers to distribute to the men sitting at the counter. Then, out of a murmur of chatter, one voice rose above the rest: "Some people are educated above their level of intelligence."

A man named Don approached me. I introduced myself and explained that I was studying the effects of living in a disease-cluster community—how people make sense of and manage illness. He didn't seem to realize I had overheard him scoffing at me. This was interesting to me because Don was a community insider who clearly didn't want to let me in and yet insisted that I interview him.

Don came to the interview on his lunch break from painting a house wearing overalls splattered with white paint. The first point that he made in our conversation was that he was a longtime resident of Clyde. "Well, I've lived in this town seventy-nine years," he said. "My family's lived here all their lives, and they go back, way back. Probably really early 1800s. It's a good town. I like everybody, I know everybody, and it's been good to me."

"Do you feel that your health is pretty good?"

"Well, I had my hand smashed, found out I got sugar, but I've been lucky. On my dad's side, all of the five kids had cancer but one. I think on my dad's side, the gene is wrong. Now my dad, he worked in dust five days a week sanding knife handles, and he got leukemia. They said it could've been from his job, but back then, there was nothin' you could do about that. Did you read the Clyde paper yesterday? Buy a Clyde paper and read the article in there that a guy put in about that cancer study—big ad. See what *he* says. He was born and raised here in Clyde. He says benzaldehyde is in food, perfume, hair spray—it's in *everything*. Now I don't know how these people can say that it got in their attic from Whirlpool. The same guy wrote an article a few weeks ago about the orchards here. This whole area years ago was surrounded by orchards. Everywhere. And they all sprayed. When you went by on the road, you could see the spray runnin' out of a wagon, going up in the air. They've been doin' it for a hundred years. Clyde had a lot of factories that are not there anymore, but they never bring them up. They never bring them up. They're gone, burnt down. I don't wanna get involved. If they have ten more meetings, I'm not going. I just don't like the idea that they're blaming it on the Whirlpool Park, like PCBs."

Don was referring to the recent discovery of nine feet of toxic sludge of PCBs under the basketball court at the former Whirlpool Park.

"The class after me . . . I don't know how many's had cancer, but a whole mess. Probably close to 50 percent. But *that's* never come out. In fact, the house I'm working on right now, his wife was in that class and she died of cancer. I talked to him about it this morning. He said it was such a rare cancer that they didn't even think there was any of that in this area, whatever she died of." Although he didn't want to attach responsibility to Whirlpool, Don was confirming suspicions about toxic contamination and the rates of cancer existing within the community even prior to the formal public health assessment that had been conducted.

"What stands out for you when you think about the first time that you heard that toxins might be causing illness in the community?"

"Well I mean, I feel sorry for the people. It's hard when you lose a kid, but I just can't see Whirlpool . . . there's been nobody at Whirlpool Park more than I've been in Whirlpool Park. I hunted it every October for duck. But I'll say one thing, everybody used that park. It was full all the time. But uh . . . I . . . and a lot of people think that they're goin' about it the wrong way. A couple of weeks ago, there's a guy down there now, very big guy, my cousin—he told Warren he was barkin' up the wrong tree." Don was referencing Warren Brown, whose daughter Alexa died from a brain tumor. Alexa's diagnosis caught the attention of residents in the community—friends and acquaintances alike expressed shock when they learned that she had cancer. Alexa would become the face of the childhood cancer cluster.

"Boy, ol' Warren, he went off the handle and he hasn't been in here much since. That was two weeks ago, but John said, 'You can't blame it on Whirlpool' . . . ya know, that's what John said. But Warren said, 'Well I ain't givin' up until I find out what killed my daughter!' And I can understand that part. . . . I just wish . . . I do know a lot of the people that are suin' for money. Not *all* of them, but a lot of 'em. Well, if Whirlpool would leave, this county would die. My house would be worth $20,000 if Whirlpool would ever leave. They employ over 3,000 people!"

This wasn't an exaggeration. Whirlpool employs nearly half of the town. Don's compassion for the families seemed genuine, but it conflicted with the impacts of Whirlpool leaving. He credited the town's economic prosperity with the establishment of the company.

"And I, when I just come in, my cousin was settin' up there at the bar. Well, he just got the word—not good. Cancer. But it . . . I don't know if it's bad here or everywhere. I mean, I don't know. I don't know if Whirlpool trips the genes or what, but, uh, I think it's O.L.D. down there, north of town—that was a disaster for Clyde. Ohio Liquid Disposal. But they had a class action suit. We won. I settled for $324. I lived on the edge and the people that lived right there got thousands and thousands."

Don was referring to a facility located just north of Clyde in Vickery, Ohio, that currently operates four Class I hazardous underground injection wells used to dispose of liquid industrial wastes and hazardous wastes generated off-site by other companies. Three other wells at the facility have been plugged and abandoned.

The injection well, formerly known as the Ohio Liquid Disposal ("O.L.D."), site, was at the center of a class action lawsuit first filed in 1983. In what the court described as a multifaceted complaint, the most salient points of that complaint alleged that the dump site operators were involved in the negligent "transportation, receipt, storage, and disposal of toxic, poisonous, hazardous, and disease-causing chemical substances."[1] The Ohio Supreme Court affirmed both the court of appeals and trial courts' decision that plaintiff-appellees be certified as a class, stating that "a class of people within five miles of the Vickery, Ohio facility suffered serious and debilitating emotional distress due to the operation of the facility."[2] While official court records are not extant, a settlement was possibly reached, as residents recall being compensated based on their proximity to the site.

Don continued, "Overall this town can't be beat. If you wanna work in this town, there's work. All my friends and everybody, they love Clyde. But we got everything because of Whirlpool. I mean the city income tax—what a wealthy town! I mean it's just that, ya know, it's the town of Whirlpool."

Although the profitability of Whirlpool likely translated into tax dollars that improved the community, Clyde hardly appeared to be wealthy—vacant storefronts occupied the downtown area. The downtown felt as if it held quite a bit of history; the vacancies make the whole street feel as if it's not fulfilling its purpose.

"And if there was somebody in dire need that ever needed somethin', this town comes out by the hundreds. We just had a fundraiser three or four weeks ago. The boy, he's forty-seven, he got Lou Gehrig's disease. Had a chicken barbecue, 1,500 chickens. They sold 'em out in a couple weeks. I don't know why God lets 'em get sick. . . . I just, well, I really think it's just an act of God. That's my own personal thinking. When it's ever settled, it'll just go back to little old Clyde. I mean, overall about the town and everything you probably won't find out any more than what I told ya."

I thanked Don for the interview. We parted ways and he returned to the house he was painting. As I drove out of Clyde, I reflected on the community as an industry town and its long history of cancer and toxic industry. I also thought about Don's reluctance to blame Whirlpool for the discovery of toxins at the park, and how the normative loyalty that people like Don have to their hometowns affect what they define as reality, what is opted or excluded from it, and how we respond emotionally to it.

A BRIEF HISTORY OF CLYDE, OHIO

The Industrial Revolution of the eighteenth and nineteenth centuries involved technological, socioeconomic, and cultural changes that transformed a once agrarian culture into a modern, streamlined society. After the conclusion of the

Civil War, Ohio evolved into a heavily industrialized state largely due to the natural attributes of the Great Lakes and river systems, which supported import and export shipping for iron ore and other products. An infrastructure of railroads supported the transport of goods and people throughout the state.[3] The population expansion paralleled rapid industrialization, as the appeal of job opportunities attracted hundreds of thousands of immigrants.[4]

Many early factories were developed to meet the demands of agriculture, producing farm machinery or processing farm products. As the need for machinery increased, Ohio's industrial importance to American economic growth came to be exemplified by companies such as the Hopewell Furnace company, an iron manufacturing facility established in 1804 and located near Youngstown, Ohio, and others. The development of these companies established northeast Ohio as the primary region for steel production by the end of the nineteenth century.[5] Development of the steel industry advanced with the discovery of coal deposits, leading to Ohio's ranking as the second-largest steel-producing state after Pennsylvania. Other natural resources also contributed to the state's industrial growth, including natural gas, oil, salt, iron ore, timber, and limestone. The Dow Chemical Company was established in Cleveland in 1895. In 2017, it merged with DuPont and was later spun off by its parent company, Dow Inc. Today Dow Inc. is among the three largest chemical producers in the world.[6]

Within archives about this area, there are two stories of its early settlers discovering springs of water that became highly valued for their healing properties. In the late nineteenth century, Thomas Dewey, the owner of two farms approximately one mile west of Clyde, was "fortunate enough to strike a mineral fountain spring . . . , the water possessing great healing and medicinal properties. It is highly valued by the people of this vicinity, who resort to it in large numbers to drink of and secure supplies of this valued water."[7] Green Springs, the town adjacent to Clyde, is known for having the largest natural sulfur spring in the world. It acquired its name from the emerald-rich color of the water produced by the sulfur and other minerals contained within it. The overflow runs into Green Creek and eventually into Sandusky Bay and Lake Erie. In the early nineteenth century, the first water-powered sawmill and grist mills were established there, which attracted many new settlers to the area.[8] The springs were reputed to possess highly curative medicinal properties, and people from many parts of Ohio came to be near the water. As part of a national trend of the time, the mineral water was also bottled and sold throughout the country for its medicinal qualities.[9] This contributed to the attraction of this area as being both wholesome and idyllic and was integral to its bucolic identity.

Clyde began its transition into a more industrialized town in the late nineteenth century with the emergence of new manufacturing businesses. In the 1890s, Clyde—like the nearby cities of Cleveland and Toledo—joined the automobile revolution. It hosted a brass-era company until the company was bought

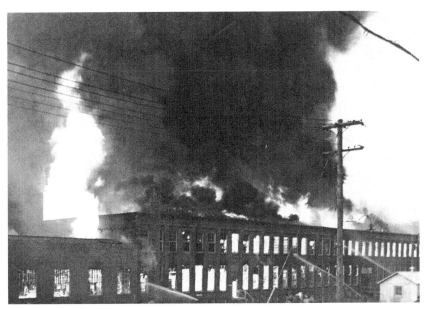

FIGURE 1. "Clyde Porcelain Steel Fire, Clyde, Ohio." 1945. Hale's Portrait Studio, Clyde, Ohio. (Courtesy of the Clyde Museum of the Clyde Heritage League.)

out by General Motors and became defunct in 1912.[10] Clyde Cutlery was established in 1904, and at one time employed over 200 workers.[11] The company remained in business until a fire destroyed the manufacturing division in 1970. Other early industries included the Hughes Granite & Marble Company and Clyde's Silver Fleece Kraut Company. Prior to 1945, Clyde Porcelain Steel Corporation was the village's biggest industry. Between 800 and 1,000 people worked at the plant, which manufactured end connectors for tanks and spark arresters for the government.[12] It burned down in 1945 and was then rebuilt (see Figure 1).

In 1952, the Whirlpool manufacturing company purchased the 250,000-square-foot facility from Clyde Porcelain Steel. Two years later, Whirlpool purchased an adjacent 170,000-square-foot facility from Bendix Corporation, a washing machine maker. With gradual expansions the factory slowly grew to its current size and is today a 240-acre campus in Clyde. The building itself is a sprawling facility of 2.4 million square feet, the equivalent of fifty-five football fields. Whirlpool Corporation's Clyde Division is the largest automatic washing machine plant in the world.[13]

Sandusky County Economic Development Corporation (SCEDC) has assisted this company in various ways, including facilitating tax incentives and, more specifically, through the recruitment of potential suppliers to this community, with the development of a skilled and available workforce, and through facilitating relationships with state and local governments.[14] As a result, Whirlpool

Corporation has provided economic stability to the town, and changed the identity from a diversely employed community to that of a factory town. From its beginning, the company has woven itself into the civic and social fabric of the town as well, and in 1953, it built a twenty-seven-acre recreational park, Whirlpool Park, in Green Springs. This park was donated to the community for recreational use and included a one-acre pool, tennis and basketball courts, and family picnic facilities. This family-friendly space was open to relatives and friends of Whirlpool workers, providing a source of entertainment. The company also promoted the notion of "family values" within its entire communications structure, advancing the case for taking a seat at the family table.

Whirlpool Corporation employs about 3,000 residents from Clyde, which has a population of approximately 6,350 residents, and the surrounding area.[15] With the manufacturing industry employing residents at over three times the average of other areas, unemployment in Clyde is consistently lower than the Ohio state average. Approximately 89.9 percent of the population is white, 6.8 percent Hispanic or Latinx, and 0.0 percent Asian. The Black population (1.0 percent) and the "foreign-born" population (0.0 percent) were significantly below the state average. Length of residence since moving is above the state average—a point reinforced by many interview participants, who told me that most people who grow up in Clyde tend to live in or close to Clyde as adults to have their own families. The median household income in Clyde is $50,054, about $8,000 less than the state median level. Approximately 11.7 percent of residents hold a college degree, which is much lower than the state average of 28.9 percent.[16] Clyde is a working-class town with its fortunes tied to Whirlpool.

SCOPE OF THE BOOK

This book focuses on community responses to residential toxic exposure in the small town of Clyde, Ohio, where a disproportionate number of children have been diagnosed with or have died of cancers of the brain and central nervous system. There exist many cases of citizen-led action that followed the sudden discovery of toxic threat.[17] More recently, scholars have directed their attention to cases of communities where little or no collective mobilization occurs.[18] I examine how economic vulnerability merges with constructed perceptions of community identity to suppress the emergence of collective action. Community inaction in the face of potential or established environmental harm warrants attention because such cases are becoming more common and more difficult to explain.[19] Why, when encountering threat to the health of so many children (and many adults too), would anyone choose to stand down? What prevents some from challenging the status quo while others contest it?

With the rise of environmental hazards worldwide, an understanding of agency in contaminated communities is increasingly important. In recent history, environmental regulation has arguably become the most vulnerable it has been in the United States since the establishment of the U.S. Environmental Protection Agency. Industry-backed politicians have overseen drastic reductions in corporate spending on pollution control and remediation.

Using the example of Clyde, Ohio, this book explores how communities navigate environmental risk and embodied risk. How does risk present discursively and what functions does it serve? How are social and political responses to toxic risk influenced and reproduced through social habits and cultural circumstances? How do social inequalities shape residents' experiences of risk? To begin to answer these questions, I use open-ended, in-depth interviews with forty Clyde residents about environmental contamination and community, along with archival documents to address the above questions. I examine a narrative wherein emotions ultimately worked to protect a company suspected of contaminating the community in which it operated. I demonstrate how emotion contributes to social hierarchies and plays a part in hampering efforts to effect social change.

This book enriches existing agendas in environmental sociology and the sociology of emotion in several ways. First, it serves to bring a critical cultural analysis of emotion from the margins to the center in the disasters literature. Sociologists have challenged conventional ideas that emotions are innate or universal responses to external occurrences—a model driven by psychologists. In recent years, there has been an upsurge of interest in emotion among sociologists. In his American Sociological Association presidential address, Eduardo Bonilla-Silva called on sociologists and policymakers to advance theories of racialized emotions—to understand their collective nature and how they function. Environmental sociologists have also been studying how emotion operates in relation to community engagement with environmental issues. As environmental anthropologist Peter Little observes, "What is at stake in spaces of toxics contamination and mitigation is how life politics are negotiated and how emotions—the affect of life politics—are constantly in-the-making; reconfigured in response to new situations, new zones of intersubjective practice, new spaces of ambiguity."[20] Building on this scholarship, this book examines the social dimensions of pride, shame, and fear and how they interact to suppress collective action. Sites of environmental conflict provide an excellent opportunity to explore dynamics of power because they are sites of social tension that are rich with affective value.

Second, this book builds on a growing body of environmental sociological research that appreciates assumptions inherent to culture as a central factor in our explanations of civic responses to environmental issues.[21] Scholars from a wide range of disciplines have studied meaning-making, pointing to cultural, rather than individual, factors that influence the ways people make judgments, including judgments about risk.[22] Sociologists have questioned the dichotomy and the hierarchy between emotion and reason in understanding and grappling with environmental crises. Individual and civic engagement on such issues cannot be grasped solely through an individualist, rationalist lens that ignores the complex tangle of meanings and feelings that influence environmental decision making and sociocultural relationships.[23]

My research points to not only a fear driven by economic anxiety but also a fear of losing security within the community—a sort of pride that is about not only status, but connectedness. While focusing on environmental risk and embodied risk, each of which occupy their own analytical space, my research indicates a social form of risk—the desire for belonging and the risk of not belonging. Risk, in this sense, occupies the space between pride (belonging) and shame (not belonging) and is very consequential to how people make judgment and respond to issues, as well as their own subjectivity.

I show how moral hierarchies and the relational processes of othering worked to preserve the town's identity and maintain the existing relationship between the town and Whirlpool. Attempts to preserve this relationship in Clyde were made as plaintiffs were met with criticism on several levels. By othering and shaming them, divisions were established, the outcome of which brought them back into the fold of community compliance. Presumptions of moral integrity that are contingent on othering are key to establishing value and valuelessness around a marginalized human population. Acknowledging "othering" not just as an outcome of this process but as integral to it opens the possibility of pinpointing the mechanisms by which social inequality is reproduced. I consider how emotions such as pride, shame, and fear contribute to this process.

Third, I push beyond looking at how social categories like race, class, and gender shape environmental justice struggles to focus on the upstream processes that produce and maintain difference in the first place. In its explicit attention to value and valuelessness, this book complements the field of critical environmental justice (CEJ), advanced by David Pellow.[24] What I bring to this is an analysis of neoliberal subjectivity that exposes how entrenched inequality is. The broader track of this book points to a major gap in government response to disease clusters, as well as the limitations of risk assessment. These barriers are a function of the broader goals of neoliberalism, which shift the burden of responsibility and self-protection onto individuals and households. I illustrate that the personal responsibility and self-protection assumed by impacted residents is an option of last resort rather than ideological commitment, which provides only a limited sense of security for those impacted by disease.

THEORETICAL FRAMEWORK

From pollution to political debates about undocumented immigrants, the notion of risk has become a central political and cultural concept that characterizes modern social life. Although the concept of risk is broad, this book deals primarily with environmental risks and embodied risks that are related to toxic exposure and its social corollaries. Risk represents the potential for loss, and like other scholars, I define risk as referring to "a situation or event where something of human value (including humans themselves) has been put at stake and where the outcome is uncertain."[25] I characterize Clyde as a "risk community" because many residents live with a heightened awareness of risk yet the toxins within the town are largely imperceptible.

Risk and subjectivity are theoretical frameworks that guide the chapters that follow. Even within the social sciences, risk has been conceptualized differently over time. The "big" theories on risk, propelled by social theorists such as Ulrich Beck and Mary Douglas, have given rise to even more complex and nuanced bodies of literature, many of which also reinforce that risk is central to human subjectivity. Much of this literature is concerned with risk perception—factors that shape risk perception, disparities in public and scientific understandings of risk, and how people judge the acceptability of risks. Scholars have also documented community responses to contamination and pollution, and the psychosocial effects of toxic contamination on communities and neighborhoods.[26] Like others working in this area, I define environmental harm as not only damage to people, property, or the environment but also less quantifiable impacts such as distress, anxiety, and fear related to socio-environmental disruptions.[27]

The theoretical and conceptual frameworks that I draw from in my case study of Clyde, Ohio, are based on a range of sources, including prior research on the social production of risk and the sociology of disasters. This literature provides frameworks from which to begin thinking about what happened in this community. The cultural/symbolic perspective advanced by Mary Douglas, for example, amplifies the importance of defining an individual's social position inside or outside a bounded social group.[28] Douglas was the first to argue that cultural, rather than individual, factors influence the ways that people make judgments. From this perspective, risk is used to reproduce and maintain concepts of selfhood and group membership. Douglas writes, "When faced with estimating probability and credibility, [individuals] come already primed with culturally learned assumptions and weightings."[29] However, Douglas, as well as other theorists of risk, falls short in addressing the question of how risk functions, not only as a measure of inequality but as a mechanism of power.

There is a Foucauldian theme that underlies this book in my examination of power as both repressive and productive. I focus on how risk is a subjective phenomenon that is largely influenced or determined by social factors such as group membership and the power relations that underlie the social meanings that inform risk. This power is repressive in that it works in service of a neoliberal agenda at the expense of people's well-being. But through the creation of normative categories, it is also productive because it drives people to respond to risks in a particular way. Acknowledging "othering" not just as an outcome but as integral to processes that produce and maintain difference opens the possibility of better understanding inequality and how emotion relates to the operation of power.

A distinct, but complementary, body of scholarship on othering has become central to sociological analyses and cultural studies of how societies establish identity categories and helps answer the question of how risk is culturally constructed, as a product of social and economic systems that privilege those who "belong" over those on the margins.[30] Because meanings develop through patterns of political and cultural practices to create sense of place, it is also useful to consider how whiteness is lived as a background to the experience of community.[31]

I make a distinction between the way risk is dealt with in public forums and the subjective experience of risk in personal life. I situate culture as inhering in everyday practices of language and relationality. Reflecting a basic tenet of sociology, I maintain the premise that people work together to create and sustain social organization while preserving an explicit analysis of power.

METHODS

This research draws on fieldwork conducted in 2013, with subsequent interviews conducted from 2014 to 2020 in Clyde and Green Springs, Ohio, both of which lie within an identified disease cluster. The bulk of data collection was carried out in the summer of 2013 when I moved into Clyde and rented a room from a family with generational ties to the community. As a result of the class action lawsuit, community tension was high during this time, which provided a unique opportunity to explore community dynamics. I conducted forty interviews and got to know key individuals in the community, including respected longtime residents and plaintiffs. I also conducted fifteen follow-up interviews with residents during subsequent visits to the community. A purposive sampling technique was used to recruit participants. In-depth interviews were conducted with residents of Clyde and Green Springs, key neighborhood leaders, plaintiffs, Whirlpool employees, teachers, nurses, impacted families, and general residents. All interviewees were white. The interview sample highlights key impact variables, including age, length of residence, and proximity of homes to the suspected pollution source.

I engaged in participant observation by attending neighborhood meetings, community picnics, and cancer fundraising events. I also spent time observing and writing fieldnotes at various public locations throughout the community to capture participants' experiences in their "everyday lives."[32] To supplement interview and observational data, I collected information through newspapers, local meetings, government reports, and public community archival documents.

I used a semistructured guide to organize the interviews. Each interview guide consisted of approximately fifteen questions designed to capture narratives around the topics of contamination experience and community identity. Open-ended questions were asked to elicit more genuine information, and semistructured interviewing allowed participants to tell their stories in their own ways and at their own pace. Interviews ranged in length from forty minutes to two hours. Interviews were digitally recorded, transcribed, and analyzed in ATLAS.ti. Open and focused coding contributed to locating the narratives within a basic social process and finding common themes among participants' responses and connections between them.[33]

Analytic techniques included active listening, which required concentration on what the participant was saying, differentiating between the participant's "inner voice" versus his or her "public voice," and simultaneously being aware of the "process as well as the substance."[34] Although interviewees' responses were largely based on their verified personal experiences, some information was presented in the form of hearsay and cannot, as such, be verified. However, it served a rhetorical purpose in establishing the commonality of rumor and repeated anecdotal speculation. Analysis was accounted for in the form of analytical and theoretical memos. In aggregate, the interviews, participant observation, and archival research allowed for a deeper understanding of emotion and community inaction.

CHAPTER OUTLINE

In chapter 1, I outline the history of neoliberalism and how its organizing rationale has led to the decline of the welfare and regulatory state, with specific attention to chemical regulation. I examine how pollutants have been regulated over time, and more recent steps taken to clear the backlog of new chemicals awaiting EPA approval. After heavy lobbying by the chemical industry, the EPA also narrowed the scope of its risk evaluations by changing the way the federal government determines health and safety risks associated with potentially toxic chemicals, with consequences for both public health and structural support for communities living with environmental contamination.

I then turn to specifics of the U.S. EPA today and the attack on community health, exploring the logics that guide deregulation and how we got to where we are today in the post-truth, anti-science era. I discuss how, because of weakened traditional institutions intended to safeguard public welfare, citizens must rely on themselves as self-governing agents. The individualization of risk becomes a feature of personal responsibility and part of the larger ideology of neoliberal governance. I explore maternal health as being particularly vulnerable to toxins and health promotion materials that target pregnant women and mothers. I discuss scholarship on precautionary consumption as well as the gendered dimension of placing responsibility for contaminant avoidance on women, especially mothers.[35] Understanding the factors that increase physical and social vulnerability help demonstrate how environmental health risks are produced.

After providing an account of environmental risk and lax regulatory standards more generally, I turn to the topic of suspected environmental risk in Clyde, Ohio. Chapter 2 outlines the events that led to the discovery of widespread cancer in the area and documents accounts of suspected illegal dumping from local industries. I follow the struggle of affected families in getting information and help from state officials, and I examine the limitations of risk assessment in the face of scientific uncertainty regarding largely imperceptible toxins and where regulatory action is dictated by scientific proof. The conflict among various stakeholders in investigating environmental risk highlights the underlying conflict between scientific authority and moral authority. From the discovery of the cancer cluster to residents assuming the burden of proof of contamination, I show how townspeople bear the burden of personal responsibility and how they, ultimately, are unable to hold anyone accountable.

Building on classic work on communities in disaster, chapter 3 details the impact of disaster on social relationships.[36] I turn to emotions to examine the question of how risk-related discourses and strategies operated among the residents who disapproved of or were publicly critical of the lawsuit against Whirlpool for suspected contamination and elevated cancer rates. I illustrate how residents engage in emotion work by othering plaintiffs, propelling a script that residents are only "true" residents if they align themselves with the company and against those "others" who threaten the core meaning of "small town." This script draws on longer histories of articulation that are conflated with affective value around notions of family and community.

Although this chapter complements scholarship that points specifically to minority environments as being deemed appropriately polluted spaces, I approach this from a different angle—one that is informed by critical whiteness studies. The culture of Clyde and Green Springs suggests an environment that operates on the "normalization" of whiteness as a standard mechanism for moving through the world, with the presumptive advantages it entails. When benefits presumed by long-standing expectations are unmet, as occurred in Clyde, the question presents as to whether whiteness itself was an inhibiting factor that contributed to complacency in their collective response. Emotions including fear, confusion, guilt, powerlessness, and denial contribute to how the community, despite being aware of risk, minimizes threat to support the continuity of their life pattern. I demonstrate how emotion contributes to social hierarchies and plays a part in hampering efforts to effect social change.

In chapter 4, I consider emotions in examining the question of how risk-related discourses and strategies operate, how they may be taken up, negotiated, or resisted by those who are the subject of them. In contrast to an exclusively social constructionist position, I demonstrate that it is constructive to investigate the ways that risk relates to the material body. Like environmental risks, their perception of which is associated with instability and fear, embodied risks are related to a type of fear that is, at once, structurally determined and socially transformative.

In conversation with literature on the illness experience, this chapter reveals some of the unseen challenges faced by those with cancer, as well as parents and siblings of children with cancer. I consider how neoliberalism shapes the environment within which chronic illness is experienced and managed. This includes the ways in which parents and siblings experience an imbalance between the role demands placed on them and the resources at their disposal to meet those demands. In the same light, I consider self-efficacy as an affective component of the self-concept that is in part determined by the availability of and access to quality health care, paid and unpaid work, and the health of the neighborhood where one lives. Uncertainty about treatment and outcomes, coupled with external barriers to care, elevated the level of strain experienced by families by adding to their financial burden, impacting parents' ability to work, and splitting families up. The responsibility for determining how families would manage this long-distance relationship fell on the parents. These social structures affected not only parents' sense of control but also their mental health, as their sense of helplessness challenged one of the primary roles of parenthood, that of being able to protect their children.

Despite the financial and emotional burden borne by families, these outcomes of an underfunded health-care system that downloads the costs to the individual are normalized. Because individuals are unable to bear this burden of health care that is available at a cost so prohibitive as to make it almost impossible for people to actually access, the community steps in to help. In this particular circumstance, fundraisers—viewed in the most positive light—are a way for communities to share resources, to support each other, and to build community. But the community creates boundaries around this resource-sharing, and while fundraising is largely laudable, it too comes with its own burdens. Impacted families, sometimes conveying feelings of disconnection, expressed a desire for an understanding of their struggles.

For those with embodied risk, awareness of risk has penetrated the (emotional) dialogue of everyday life, often merging with notions of personal responsibility for risk protection. Within a context where the imperative for self-protection is impossible to achieve, impacted families experience psychosocial and practical conflicts as they adapt to cancer as a way of life.

I conclude with chapter 5, which reflects on what some call the "post-truth era" and culminates in a more complete understanding of how risk is reproduced through social and political processes. I consider the important role of grassroots activists in empowering residents who are fighting toxic threats, and in bringing creative strategies to guide their resistance. I also reflect on the mutual benefits of academic and grassroots collaboration. Considering a future where debates about risk and science will inevitably increase, I consider possibilities for the democratization of risk management and the need for transformative approaches to environmental justice—namely, a reconceptualization of body and environment.

The people of Clyde had to navigate a complex social and economic situation while also dealing with the loss of their children. Often, in the aftermath of disaster, fault lines emerge between the affected and unaffected in a way that reproduces preexisting structural inequalities and corrodes attitudes of unity. There were powerful incentives for preserving the Whirlpool connection—not just preserving the source of employment for much of the town but protecting a long-cherished community identity as well. Increasing industrial influence on safety assessments of chemicals threatens community health, generates confusion, and can result in literally no response equal to the gravity of problems faced by contaminated communities.

1 ▸ THE DEREGULATION OF TOXIC CHEMICALS

NEOLIBERALISM AND THE DECLINE OF THE WELFARE AND REGULATORY STATE

Composed of a transnational network of neoliberals, the Mont Pelerin Society was formed in 1947 to promote the market as a central agent in society, thereby shifting government focus from public welfare to market creation and protection.[1] In the post–Cold War era of the United States, Ronald Reagan was a critical influence in fostering changes that transformed neoliberal theory into reality. The neoliberal ethos combines a commitment to individual liberty with the economic ideas of the free market and an opposition to state intervention in that market. A central logic of neoliberalism is that decentralized efforts of individual entrepreneurs and firms operating in free markets will create more jobs and income than any collective action. Neoliberal thinking has come to dominate many influential institutions including think tanks and has become the dominant philosophy of international financial institutions such as the World Bank and the International Monetary Fund, prompting its spread to the global economic system, where nations are enmeshed in webs of social, economic, and cultural interdependence.

The globalization of the production process breaks down and systematically integrates national circuits into new global circuits of accumulation. This fragmentation and decentralization, along with the spread of multinational corporations, has led to a shift in power marked by global economic management and decision making in transnational capital and its agents.[2] David Harvey argues that restoring the class power of the global economic elite is the central mission of neoliberalism.[3] Neoliberalism has elevated the position of economic elites in the United States and elsewhere across the globe at the expense of the working class, resulting in massive social inequality and environmental degradation.[4]

While neoliberal policies are unevenly implemented across the globe in different settings, proponents of neoliberalism celebrate it as elevating the standard of living for people and even creating a world culture that respects individual rights and weakens dictators.[5] As well-known scholar and neoliberal economist William Easterly argues, the empirical record on the difference between economic performance of freedom, which prioritizes the individual over the group, and that of collectivism, which emphasizes the group over the self, illustrates how free societies have dramatically outperformed collectivist ones over the last half century.[6] Easterly summarizes several reasons free markets thrive. One point is that, given the difficulty in predicting which economic actions will succeed and which will fail, relying on feedback mechanisms from markets, rather than governments, is a more efficient way to reallocate resources toward what is succeeding. Economic freedom also fosters success in finding niches in international markets wherein a country can achieve large-scale manufacturing exports. In contrast to centralized planning bureaucracies, Easterly argues, economic freedom fosters competition, leading the best to succeed and resulting in a higher standard of living.

Inherent in these points is the neoliberal critique of state reason, an important starting point for understanding how science has become commercialized. As noted by science and technology studies scholars Rebecca Lave, Philip Mirowski, and Samuel Randalls, neoliberalism is not merely a system of economic exchange; it is also the processing and conveyance of knowledge and information to "alter the ontology of the market, and consequently, to revise the very conception of society."[7] Connecting the limits of government to the inherent limitations on a state's power to know and therefore to supervise promotes the market as the best at processing information.[8] This enables the political strategy of the neoliberal network to promote capitalism by reducing the role of governments in the regulation of national economies.

Aside from debates on taxation and redistribution, it is the "regulatory state"—the set of laws, rules, and institutions set up to govern the economy and society—that most influences the degree of freedom held by a country's market economy. In advanced industrial societies like the United States, the state's role in developing, monitoring, and enforcing market rules has been reduced through policy and in its institutions, while industries have been given a great deal of freedom to self-regulate. Yet stemming from the idea that competition always prevails is a neoliberal logic that corporations can do no wrong and should not be blamed if they do. Furthermore, as noted by Lave, Mirowski, and Randalls, "the market (suitably re-engineered and promoted) can always provide solutions to problems seemingly caused by the market in the first place"—monopoly is eventually undone by "competition"; pollution is abated by the trading of "emissions permits."[9]

Despite its continual encroachment upon policy, cultural ideology, and even our own subjectivity, two assumptions in the capitalist logic create ongoing tensions for neoliberalism: the steady accumulation of wealth by capitalists will improve the conditions for all of society, and the world's resources are infinite.[10] Social movements scholar Jackie Smith observes that the blatant falsehood of these assumptions requires the neoliberal network to continually work to defend its positions. The commercialization of science has enabled subsequent attacks on science, a neoliberal movement directed at the intentional obfuscation of those tensions. Examining the history of chemicals and their regulation is important for understanding the influence of neoliberalism on policy and provides a window into science commercialization.

CHEMICAL DEREGULATION IN THE UNITED STATES

The chemical industry is composed of companies that produce industrial chemicals by converting raw materials such as fossil fuels, minerals and metals, and water into products. Most chemical companies are also plastic manufacturers. The inceptions of major U.S. chemical companies, including DuPont, Monsanto, Union Carbide, and Dow Chemical, were rooted in the production of weaponry and war materials beginning prior to World War I.[11] By-products of explosives were later used to develop insecticides.[12] The production of polyvinyl chloride (PVC), polystyrene, and polyethylene, developed before World War II, contributed to increased demand for new, lightweight products to be used for a variety of items ranging from weaponry to food packaging. When, at the conclusion of the war, attention was directed toward marketing plastic goods to the American public, lucrative possibilities for the chemical industry expanded. After World War II, as engineers developed increasingly diverse plastic products, chemical companies looking for new avenues for production employed strategic advertising to alter their wartime image to that as manufacturers of more utilitarian and beneficial products.[13] Companies such as Dow, Monsanto, and DuPont launched extensive advertising campaigns that promoted the modern versatility of their products with a focus on manufacturing plastic goods for use in postwar households, allowing for capitalization of the country's rapid economic growth (see Figure 2).[14] "Better things for better living . . . through chemistry" was the DuPont motto used to define the burgeoning industry.[15]

Today the industry produces a wide variety of products that are components of or are required in manufacturing processes for nearly every consumer

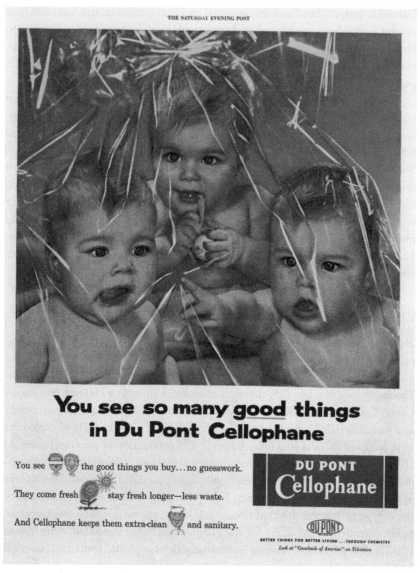

FIGURE 2. Advertisement for Du Pont Cellophane from the *Saturday Evening Post*, 1955. (Courtesy of the Hagley Museum and Library.)

and industrial product. Because of how frequently chemicals are combined with other chemicals in synthetic processes, chemical company customers are often other chemical companies.[16] Although the proliferation of plastic products made consumer goods readily available to the average American and provided more equitably affordable conveniences, it also infiltrated homes with thousands of unregulated chemicals that had potentially deleterious effects on the health of people using them.[17] These products, although potentially harmful, were happily integrated into the vast catalog of consumer items by an unsuspecting public that assumed safety measures were in place when, in fact, such measures were neither taken nor able to be so. Concern for long-term effects and consequences on people's health and the environment was negligible as the unbridled drive to produce salable goods increased profit margins to extraordinary levels.

As early as the 1950s, scientists and lawmakers were becoming aware of public health risks associated with unregulated chemicals. Early documentation indicates unwillingness and subterfuge on the part of chemical companies in releasing findings regarding potentially harmful chemicals to the public.[18] During the same time that the U.S. Congress attempted to intervene and protect consumers by writing legislation that would require the study of adverse health effects of chemicals used in food and cosmetics, a committee led by Congressman James T. Delaney introduced three amendments: the Pesticide Amendment (1954), the Food Additives Amendment (1958), and the Color Additive Amendment (1960).[19] These amendments significantly changed the U.S. food and drug law. With them, no substance could be legally introduced into the U.S. food supply unless it had been predetermined to be safe, placing the burden of that determination on manufacturers.[20] However, these attempts to regulate chemicals were met with strong opposition from a powerful, influential chemical industry whose promotion of plastic in the media not only emphasized its popularity and benefit to postwar society but also encouraged consumer trust in science and technology. By using their own scientists to refute data identifying the toxicity of their products and/or discredit proponents of chemical regulation, the chemical industry was able to redirect the outcome by obfuscating contradictory information.[21] Subsequently, when the Food Additives Bill of 1958 was passed, existing chemicals that had never been proven to be safe were grandfathered in as being safe. The consequence of this inaction allowed for the introduction of dangerous chemicals directly into households, an egregious action that threatened the sanctity and expectation of safe dwelling the unsuspecting public aspired to achieve.

In the early 1970s, the environmental movement helped to raise public awareness of toxins. Attempts at congressional regulation were again initiated, this time centered on allowing the EPA to examine chemical use and toxicity. The Toxic Substances Control Act (TSCA) of 1976 authorized the EPA to control chemicals that posed an unreasonable risk to human health or the environment. But strong lobbying and PR advertising by the chemical industry reduced the impact of the legislation as it again permitted the continued use of existing chemicals without any evaluation. The TSCA Inventory contains 87,000 chemicals that have been approved for commercial use, of which 41,864 are active. Furthermore, the statute did not give the EPA authority to reevaluate existing chemicals, nor did it give the agency authority to force companies to provide toxicity data.[22] More than 60,000 commercial chemicals were allowed on the market without safety testing.

Legally, chemical manufacturers and importers are responsible for evaluating and classifying each chemical produced in or imported by their workplaces. They are responsible for determining the hazard classes, and, where appropriate, the category of each class that applies to the chemical being classified.[23] Employers, those that employ the chemicals in use, are not required to classify chemicals unless they choose not to rely on the classification performed by the chemical manufacturer or importer to satisfy this requirement. Chemical manufacturers, importers, or employers classifying chemicals are obligated to identify and consider the full range of available scientific literature and other evidence concerning the potential hazards—there is no requirement to test the chemical to determine how to classify its hazards.

The Frank R. Lautenberg Chemical Safety for the 21st Century Act addresses fundamental flaws in TSCA that have limited EPA's ability to protect the public from harmful chemicals. Some important improvements to chemical regulation enacted by this legislation, which was passed in 2016, include requiring the EPA to evaluate the safety of existing chemicals in commerce, requiring risk-based chemical assessments, and increasing the public transparency of chemical information by limiting unwarranted claims of confidentiality. Yet limitations in the evaluation of chemicals and risk-based chemical assessments remain. One of the most important limitations to current legal rules is that when classifying mixtures they produce or import, chemical manufacturers and importers of mixtures may rely on the information provided on the current safety data sheets of the individual ingredients.[24] In other words, when testing or evaluating chemicals for their potential danger to human health or determining acceptable limits of exposure, the U.S. regulatory system considers them in isolation from each other and does not account for the transformation of these compounds via interaction. The TSCA does not list chemical mixtures; the individual components of mixtures are listed separately. This approach affords flexibility to processors, who are allowed to make many different mixtures of Inventory-listed substances without filing a Premanufacture Notice.[25] Many chemical products are intermediates—substances generated by one step and used for a subsequent step in the development of synthetic processes, and therefore numerous mixtures are created. In other words, those 60,000 untested commercial chemicals on the market are then added together in innumerable combinations that are then themselves entirely untested.

Loose campaign finance rules make it difficult to track the exact amount of money chemical companies have spent on lobbying, but finance spending based on data from the Senate Office of Public Records demonstrates an increase in lobbying when new pieces of legislation to develop stronger restrictions are introduced. The American Chemistry Council hires multiple lobbying firms, each with its own team of lobbyists who seek to influence politicians on issues that could affect their revenue. U.S. chemical industry lobbyists heavily borrow from tactics used by the tobacco industry and oil lobbies to undermine and distort the compelling scientific evidence that demonstrates the harms of chemicals to health. In addition to using strategic public relations approaches, the chemical industry exerts its commercial interests within science and medicine.

Collaboration between industry and academia is a growing phenomenon within the chemical industry. Until 1980, the federal government retained the intellectual property rights of anything produced with federal funds. Changes in patent laws embodied in the Bayh-Dole Act allow researchers (at universities and at biotech companies) funded by federal agencies to patent their discoveries and then license those patents to companies, which encourages commercialization of new technologies.[26] Providing universities with patent rights to certain inventions arising out of government-sponsored research and development has reduced companies' research costs. Industry-academia collaboration also generates innovation in the chemical and drug industry. Universities, which generally do not have the means to translate research into marketable products, are incentivized to collaborate because this work is accomplished as part of the education curriculum and provides training for scientists and engineers, some of whom then go on to work in the private sector. University researchers also receive royalty payments. Among other critiques, however, these collaborations have been criticized for creating improper conflicts of interest. In relation to the biotechnology and pharmaceutical industries, there is concern that researchers have a vested interest in emphasizing the benefits of new drugs.[27]

With increased state and federal funding cuts to public universities, universities are increasingly turning to the private sector for assistance. One example is the partnerships between Monsanto, one of the world's leading producers of genetically modified organisms, with several public universities. By 2010, private donations from corporations made up nearly one-quarter of the money used for agricultural research in land-grant universities across the United States.[28] Industry funding for research by university-based scientists has also increased since 1980 in the form of grants and all-expenses-paid conferences. In the past, university-based drug researchers provided a partial check on the drug research process by bringing a more objective eye to their research. The rollback in public funding for universities, including the National Institutes of Health and the National Science Foundation, coupled with the expectation by university administrators that faculty seek external funding, have encouraged academics to seek industry collaboration. But when industries fund university-based research, they often retain the rights to the research results. This can keep university researchers from publishing any data suggesting the ineffectiveness or danger of the chemical or drug. And while the industry has increased its funding to university-based researchers, it has even more dramatically increased funding to commercial research organizations, which are paid not only to conduct research but also to promote it. When industry controls the creation, analysis, and review of toxicological data related to new chemicals, the health effects of a chemical can be skewed to the industry's viewpoint.[29]

When science becomes commercialized through neoliberal policies that affect scientific practice and management, such as encouraging private funding for public researchers, it also becomes more easily privatized.[30] Lave, Mirowski, and Randalls importantly point out that the redefinition of property rights is also the most effective way to establish privatization programs that had previously been subject to communal or other forms of allocation.[31] Companies control data by defining them as intellectual property to both shape the interpretation of those data and to gain commercial value from knowledge.[32]

Alongside 1980s legal changes reflecting both the increasingly "business-friendly" atmosphere in the federal government and the increased influence of industry lobbying, chemical trade also began to prosper. The industry has benefited from a strong chemical trade surplus—more exports than imports—which has significantly increased since the mid-1980s.[33] In 2019, the United States had a trade surplus of $35 billion in industrial chemicals, with the largest national markets for chemical exports being Mexico and Canada.[34] Today, the United States continues to be the world's largest producer of chemicals, and the chemical industry plays an important role in the global economy. It is an enormous—and enormously profitable—enterprise. When factoring in chemicals used in pharmaceuticals, global sales totaled around $6 trillion in 2019, making the chemical industry the second largest manufacturing industry in the world.[35] Over the three years from 2021 to 2024, the industry is expected to grow in every segment, with overall industry growth expected to be 1.8 percent in 2024.[36]

The last quarter of the twentieth century was marked by growth in the commercialization of scientific knowledge, leading to changes in the production and dissemination of knowledge. The proliferation of market-oriented ideas and practices has also led to changes in the status of claims about knowledge. In the broadest sense, this is the idea that the market "knows best" and that knowledge itself can be commercialized. These changes have ultimately paved the way for dismantling institutions that rely on science and data to inform decisions on environmental and human health.

THE DISMANTLING OF ENVIRONMENTAL REGULATIONS

New policy imperatives in the 1980s, such as those created to address environmental justice and regulate pollutants like mercury and greenhouse gases, expanded the EPA's mission and responsibilities. "Deadline and hammer" amendments to the Clean Water Act and other laws, the Clean Air Act Amendments of 1990, and the Safe Drinking Water Act required the EPA to meet statutory deadlines pertaining to making safe use determinations. Yet, at the same time, the agency also faced budgeting and staffing cuts that have reduced its capacity to maintain and improve environmental quality.[37]

In addition to these setbacks that weakened the EPA, the agency has faced partisanship that has impeded new environmental statutes. When the Clean Air Act, the federal law that regulates air emissions, became law in 1970, the Senate passed it without a single nay vote. At the signing ceremony, President Richard Nixon stated, "We signed a historic piece of legislation that put us far down the road toward a goal that Theodore Roosevelt, 70 years ago, spoke eloquently about: a goal of clean air, clean water, and open spaces for the future generations of America."[38] In the years that followed, environmental policy received bipartisan support, with Republicans advocating for amendments to strengthen environmental policies to protect public health and public welfare and to expand regulation of emissions of hazardous air pollutants. But coinciding with the rise of neoliberalism, the early 1980s marked the beginning of an effort by conservatives to adjust the interpretation and enforcement of environmental laws and regulations. In response to complaints by the steel, automobile, and utilities and chemicals industries that the clean air regulations were costly and difficult to comply with, many conservatives began to distance themselves from environmentalism. While acknowledging the support for the agency from several Republican presidents, some EPA employees have pinpointed a turning point in 1994 when Republicans took over the House, which "emboldened the industry to try to interfere with the enforcement process more than ever before."[39] In 1995, Congress did not renew the Superfund tax on chemical and petroleum industries, which had served as the agency's main source of income, outside of congressional appropriations.

Thus, for regulatory agencies like the EPA that specify regulatory statutes and punish noncompliance, the decline in resources has limited the state's capacity to shape political outcomes. In the decade prior to the Obama administration, a new antienvironmental strain of neoliberal conservatism funded by Republican business elites was gaining institutional influence. The Heritage Foundation and the Competitive Enterprise Institute, American conservative and libertarian think tanks founded in the 1970s and 1980s that have received significant funding from the energy and chemical industries, turned their attention toward discrediting the growing international consensus among scientists about the impact of human activities on climate change. Like chemical industry lobbyists working from the playbooks of the tobacco industry's disinformation campaigns, a key strategy of these think tanks has been to discount science.

THE ATTACK ON COMMUNITY HEALTH

When neoliberal regimes threaten and erode democratic political institutions, communities become vulnerable. The negative impact of toxic chemicals on health is well documented. Synthetic chemicals are now present in all human bodies.[40] They are found in our environment, in our food, and in consumer products.

There is reason to believe that certain chemicals cause certain types of cancer. Naphthalene, for example, is a solid chemical commonly found in coal, mothballs, and the manufacturing of polyvinyl chloride. Manufacturing, industrial releases, improper disposal of industrial waste, and consumer use can release naphthalene into the environment. Naphthalene exposure can cause dizziness, confusion, nausea, and vomiting. It can also kill red blood cells, causing anemia. Studies in animals have shown that breathing naphthalene-contaminated air can cause nose and lung tumors. Because of this, the U.S. Department of Health and Human Services and the International Agency for Research on Cancer have both concluded that naphthalene likely causes cancer in humans.

Polychlorinated biphenyls (PCBs) are a group of human-made chemicals that were used in industrial and commercial settings for their properties as electrical insulators. Despite their ban in 1979, PCBs are still released into the environment today through poorly maintained hazardous waste sites, leaks from electrical equipment, and accidental or deliberate dumping of PCB waste. PCBs are classified by the EPA as probable human carcinogens, and exposure to PCBs has been linked to cancers such as melanoma, non-Hodgkin's lymphoma, breast cancer, and liver cancer. Exposure to PCBs also has non-cancer health effects including immune system suppression, deficits in learning and neurological development, and reproductive system effects such as decreased birth weight and birth defects. In Minden, West Virginia, the company Shaffer Equipment poured PCB-containing liquid into the ground, stored fluid in waste containers that later leaked, and sprayed PCB oils on roads to combat dust. More than 30 percent of residents have been diagnosed with cancer.[41]

Decades of scholarship demonstrates that low-income and Black communities across the country bear a disproportionate health burden from industrial pollution due to environmental racism.[42] On average, the level of cancer risk from industrial air pollution in majority-Black census tracts is more than double that of majority-white tracts.[43] Minority communities experience higher exposures to contaminants, occupy crowded living spaces, often have lower-paying, more hazardous jobs, and have economic challenges and lower access to health care. Government agencies have also been criticized for their slow response in providing relief to contaminated communities of color and imposing lower fines on companies that pollute in Black communities.

Hazardous substances are often found in higher levels in the workplace than in the general environment. Exposure to occupational and environmental carcinogens in the United States disproportionately affects lower-income workers and communities, contributing to disparities in the cancer burden. While some white-collar jobs such as dentistry and chemical engineering have been associated with high rates of cancer, the working class continues to have higher rates of morbidity and mortality due to unhealthy working environments and exposure to industrial carcinogens such as asbestos, heavy metals, and chemicals.[44] Occupational studies have also revealed elevated cancer rates among rubber and plastics factory workers, painters, barbers and hairdressers, farmers, welders, asbestos workers, dye and fabric makers, miners, printers, and radiation workers.[45] Additionally, as some have suspected to be true in the Clyde cancer cluster, studies have found links between the occupational exposures of parents and consequent cancers, particularly leukemia and nervous system cancers, in their children.[46] Much has yet to be understood regarding the roles that genetics and environmental exposures play in carcinogenesis, but one recent discovery is that of germline mutations, wherein some genetic changes that increase the risk of cancer can be passed from parent to child.[47]

Pesticides and industrial chemicals, including heavy metals such as mercury and zinc, filter into ground and surface waters. Metal degreasers and dry-cleaning fluids, which have been linked to cancers in humans, are common contaminants of glacial aquifers.[48] Dioxins and dioxin-like compounds, which are frequently the by-products of industrial processes, have been linked to diabetes, reproductive and developmental problems, damage to the immune system, interference with hormones, and cancer.[49] Additionally, over half of the toxins emitted by industries are released into air.[50] The 1990 Clean Air Act requires the EPA to set standards for permissible levels of air pollutants.[51] Yet, despite progress in improving air quality, recent data from the World Health Organization show that many U.S. cities and cities across the world fail to meet air pollution guidelines.[52] Toxic and hazardous wastes that pose a major threat to health and the environment to this day continue to be frequently disposed of in illegal, insecure, and unsafe ways.[53] Ominously, toxic and hazardous wastes can also harm communities far removed from the original toxic waste sites and/or the chemical industries that produce or use them.[54]

Chemicals such as DDT, lindane, chlordane, dieldrin, aldrin, and heptachlor that have been banned for use in the United States continue to be shipped abroad, although both chlordane and heptachlor have been linked to leukemia and childhood cancers.[55] In 2019, the United States exported about $2.25 million worth of asbestos products.[56] Lead house paint, which was banned in the U.S. in 1978, is also exported to and sold in developing countries, most often without health warnings on the products.[57] Toxins are transported between states within the United States as well. For example, the current U.S. gas and oil boom is generating millions of tons of waste from fracking. Pennsylvania sends millions of gallons of its wastewater from hydraulic fracturing to Ohio, which now has more than 200 active injection wells for oil and gas waste.[58] This broad spectrum of potentially disastrous weakness in manufacture, storage, transportation, and faulty regulatory practice has converged to impose hazardous environmental consequences on communities across the globe.

REPRODUCTIVE, MATERNAL, AND CHILDREN'S VULNERABILITY TO TOXINS

Environmental health is a women's rights issue and a children's rights issue. Women are more susceptible to autoimmune conditions than men due to their higher percentage of body fat, where larger amounts of lipophilic chemicals are stored.[59] Researchers have found associations between chemical exposure and adverse pregnancy outcomes, including preterm delivery, the leading cause of perinatal mortality.[60] Because the placenta is unable to block most synthetic chemicals stored in a woman's body fat, chemicals have the ability to cause subtle damage to the developing fetus, repercussions of which may manifest in the form of behavioral and cognitive problems, as well as birth defects.[61] Up to 300 synthetic chemicals have been found in body fat and in breast milk.[62] Despite opposite claims made by the chemical industry, a 2021 study found that both legacy and current-use PFAS now contaminate breast milk, exposing nursing infants.[63] Toxic, persistent chemicals were found in all fifty samples of women's breast milk. Exposure to toxic chemicals may also impair a woman's ability to lactate and breastfeed successfully.[64] As breastfeeding has been determined to be protective against breast cancer, this illustrates how environmental contaminants can affect lifestyle choices, and in turn, affect cancer risk.

The types of cancers that develop in children and adolescents differ from those that develop in adults. Predominant types of pediatric cancers (ages 0–19) are leukemia (26 percent), cancers of the brain and central nervous system (CNS; 18 percent), and lymphoma (14 percent). Some of the cancers that develop in children are rarely seen in adults, notably those cancers that arise from embryonic cells and originate in developing tissues and organ systems.[65]

In general, the incidence of pediatric cancer is higher in industrialized countries than in developing countries, but patterns differ by cancer type.[66] Despite major treatment advances in recent decades, childhood cancer rates overall have been slightly rising for the past few decades.[67] From 1975 to 2018, the overall incidence of pediatric cancer in the United States slightly increased by an average of 0.8 percent per year.[68] Environmental factors may be responsible for some of this increase, with improved diagnosis and access to medical care over time contributing to more cases being identified and statistically included.[69] An estimated 10,590 new cancer cases and 1,180 cancer deaths were expected to occur among children (ages 0–14) in 2018.[70] Unlike many adult cancers, incidence is not consistently higher among populations with lower socioeconomic status.[71]

The most rapid periods of growth occur in utero, during infancy, and during puberty.[72] These periods of accelerated growth, which involve an increase in the number of cells in the body, are also periods of heightened sensitivity to toxic substances.[73] In addition to having higher rates of cell proliferation, which are positively correlated with an increased susceptibility to carcinogens, children have less developed detoxifying mechanisms.[74] A child's body composition, the proportion of body weight made up of fat tissue, and the distribution of fat may also have an important influence on childhood risks from pesticides.[75]

Another reason that children are more vulnerable to toxins than are adults is that some toxins, referred to as "initiators," are not capable of inducing tumors alone but are believed to require later exposure to chemical "promoters," "which further alter the genetic code governing cell reproduction."[76] Thus, exposure to toxins during childhood increases the probability that the initiated cells will be promoted through additionally necessary stages of tumor development, given that a child has a longer period of time during which exposure to promoters may occur.

Exposure to endocrine-disrupting chemicals, such as phthalates and bisphenol A, has been cited as a risk factor for early puberty.[77] Rather than being directly linked to causing cancer, endocrine-disrupting chemicals influence our health by mimicking or altering metabolic regulation. These compounds interfere with hormone production and metabolism in ways that create biological conditions that make us more susceptible to cancer and other diseases. These chemicals are used to make synthetics malleable and are found in consumer products, including children's toys, shower curtains, and water bottles, as well as pesticides, packaging, and building materials. Consequently, children are continuously exposed to low-level endocrine disruptors in their diet, drinking water, air supply, and consumer products.[78]

THE SCIENTIFIC UNCERTAINTY OF RISK ASSESSMENT

U.S. environmental policies are based on the highest "acceptable" amount of toxic exposure, rather than on avoiding harm from toxic chemicals in the first place. In contrast, the European Union (E.U.) uses a precautionary model, under which a substance needs to be proven safe before it is exposed to the public. Given the global demand for pesticides and agricultural products, however, the E.U. is under increasing pressure to conform to U.S. regulations, which are less stringent than those in Europe.[79] Specifically, the E.U. is under pressure to alter its definition, and consequently loosen its regulation of endocrine-disrupting chemicals, which interfere with hormones and are particularly dangerous to young children. Again, as a result of lobbying, the U.S. government's position largely echoes the positions taken by chemical industry groups, such as CropLife America and the American Chemistry Council, that have a vested interest in the financial implications of chemical regulation where market analysts expect revenues to grow at a compound annual growth rate of 3.3 percent from 2020 to 2027 to reach $75.54 billion by 2027.[80]

Under the current model in the United States, communities impacted by environmental contamination carry the burden of proving that a substance is dangerous, the likelihood of which is nearly impossible. In fact, there have only been a few cases that have found a likely environmental cause—the childhood leukemia cluster in Toms River, New Jersey, and the childhood leukemia cluster in Woburn, Massachusetts.

In recent decades, much of risk research has been focused on the development of methods of and procedures for risk analysis and risk management. On this end of the spectrum, most risk research—conducted by operations managers, financial analysts, and epidemiologists alike—understands risk as an entity that can be calculated using statistics and probabilities. Researchers have debated definitional differences between risks and hazards and the ambiguous meaning of risk as "uncertainty" and its limitations for quantifying risk. At the heart of many of these definitional debates are disagreements on whether to privilege subjective or objective interpretations, with objective perspectives prevailing in favor of positivist definitions and practical applications.

Knowledge about toxins and their impact on health is based on causal interpretations. Epidemiologists rely on environmental science, lifestyle factors, and biostatistics to determine whether a suspected cluster is truly evidence of an excess of cancer cases.[81] Most are determined not to be clusters, and many are believed to occur by chance. Those that are more likely to represent true clusters are usually characterized by having a large number of cases of one type of cancer, a rare type of cancer, and/or an increased number of cases of a certain type of cancer in an age group that is not usually affected by that type of cancer.[82] Historically, higher-profile cancer clusters, such as those connected to AIDS identification or the presence of asbestos, had one or more of these characteristics.

Determining whether a community has a statistically significantly higher cancer risk than the general population requires current and complete information on the incidence of disease within that community. However, many states do not have accurate tracking systems, and many do not track the full range of conditions that may be linked to toxic exposure.[83] For example, most states do not conduct systematic tracking of learning disabilities, neurological disorders such as Alzheimer's and Parkinson's, metabolic diseases like diabetes, or autoimmune disorders such as lupus. Additionally, evaluation of many substances is inhibited by a lack of data on industrial and commercial chemicals. Although the U.S. Toxics Release Inventory (TRI) established emission registers in 1986 to improve data based on chemicals, including emissions, it depends on the public and industries to report this information. Emissions data from the chemicals industry are not easily accessible. These limitations in access to data cause delays in investigations, prevent the identification of disease trends, inhibit the identification of true clusters, and reduce the number of investigations conducted by states.[84]

Studies of suspected clusters typically focus on both genetics and environment, including behavior and lifestyle. Scientifically establishing a genetic-environmental interaction requires long-term studies of large populations.[85] It is difficult to study the relationship between exposure to potentially carcinogenic substances and cancer risk in the general population because of uncertainties about exposure and the challenges of long-term follow-up. To determine whether illnesses within a community are the result of environmental toxins, epidemiologists assess exposures by measuring how much of a contaminant can be absorbed by an exposed individual, in what form, and at what rate and how much of the absorbed amount is available to produce a biological effect. All five of the following elements must be present for an "exposure pathway" to be considered complete: (1) source (where the chemical came from), (2) environmental transport (the way the chemical moves from the source to the individual), (3) point of exposure (where contact with the chemical is made), (4) route of exposure (how the chemical enters the body), and (5) people who might be exposed (those who are most likely to come into physical contact with a chemical).[86] Consequently, the risk to exposed individuals varies according to the intensity, potency, and duration of the exposure, as well as other potential factors, including exposures to other carcinogens. Levels of exposure to industrial and agricultural pollutants are difficult to assess in nonoccupational settings, in part due to the populations at risk being less clearly defined.[87] Even in the 5 to 15 percent of reported cases wherein statistical testing confirms that the number of observed cases exceeds the number of expected cases, further epidemiologic investigation almost never identifies the underlying cause of disease with confidence.[88] Current systems for identifying and classifying evidence for carcinogenicity (at every level) and risk assessment share a common constraint: the scientific complexity of the issues at hand.

Determining the causal effect of a single toxin on health is challenging because individuals are exposed to a complex mixture of carcinogenic compounds throughout their lifetimes.[89] Additionally, the "specific mechanism by which carcinogens act is often unknown."[90] As mentioned above, for example, some toxins are referred to as "initiators." They are not capable of inducing tumors alone but are believed to require later exposure to chemical "promoters," which further alter the genetic code governing cell reproduction. It is very difficult to predict exposure to the substances now presumed to be a complex mixture of initiators and promoters. It has been shown that when compounds interact with one another, toxic effects can be more harmful than those resulting from singular exposure.[91] Just as the U.S. regulatory system does not account for chemical mixtures, it also does not account for the interactions of chemicals in biological systems. Metals, for example, including arsenic, cadmium, chromium VI, beryllium, and nickel, have emerged as an important class of human carcinogens. The mechanisms responsible for metal carcinogenesis are elusive, though, partly due to the complex nature of metals' interactions in biological systems. Calcium, a nutritionally essential metal that is important for human health because of its essential role in metabolism, nerve conduction, and muscle contraction, is also important in terms of risk assessment because of potential interactions with the principal toxic metals.[92] The unwillingness to consider the effects of compounding chemicals further delays efforts toward the prevention of disease.

Contributing to the conundrum, tests of statistical significance, which are used in standard scientific practices, are not very successful in assessing the level of threat posed by carcinogens to communities because hypothesis testing has been designed to guard against the mistake of false positives.[93] Cutoffs for statistical significance, which is represented by alpha levels commonly set at 0.10, 0.05, 0.01, or 0.001 and represent the percent of time the research is willing to risk a false positive, are designed to be conservative. But conservative cutoffs for statistical significance mean that disease clusters in communities may be overlooked, and consequently, opportunities are lost for creating meaningful policy. Statistically significant differences in the rates of cancer in small communities compared with those in surrounding areas are also unlikely to be found because of small sample sizes.

Because individual communities have limited power to identify problems in cancer cluster studies, some advocate for greater participation of citizens in the production and utilization of scientific data in disease cluster investigations— what has been termed "popular epidemiology."[94] Public participation in the research processes of contaminated communities consists of both community members and stakeholders, including site owners and industry and business. Collaboration between citizens and epidemiologists with regard to identifying and resolving environmental illness patterns is important for accomplishing public health goals. The need for collaborative research is supported from a number of professional associations and regulatory institutions, including the National Institute of Environmental Health Sciences, National Institute of Allergies and Infectious Diseases, U.S. EPA, and Centers for Disease Control and Prevention (CDC).[95] The rise of social movements has also elevated lay voices, making their contributions equally valid, and has challenged traditional methods of reducing uncertainty to the point of making risks manageable.[96] However, while popular epidemiology may be a promising path forward, it is not yet a widely used method. Even when it is used, not all communities achieve successful outcomes with regard to both collaboration and identifying causes of disease. Pessimism generated by the lack of receptiveness of government institutions leads to suspicions that the government only pays lip service to the open-ended process of public inclusion in participatory processes of discovery.[97] This attaches a moral dimension to issues of responsibility, justice, and fairness. Even in cases including public participation, victims remain largely unheard and marginalized, with governmental agents only listening to expert voices.[98] These outcomes reinforce the value of including soft sciences for the anticipation of concerns such as communication and voice-receptive agency, lay participation, and democratization of risk management.

THE GOVERNMENT OF THE SELF:
THE INDIVIDUALIZATION OF RISK AND HEALTH

Neoliberal governance has changed how people conceptualize and deal with risk. To some degree, the general public has come to tacitly accept chemical deregulation in the places once assumed to be safe. To understand how so many have bought into this state of being is to recognize that among the principles of neoliberalism, market exchange is an ethic itself and freedom is redefined as being constituted in autonomous self-governed individuals.

Foucault, who is known for his historical studies of institutions, gives us a way of understanding governmentality—how the modern state exercises individualization techniques to exert power over the subjectivity of the person. In contrast to a monarchy, where the power of the queen or king was absolute and power was imposed from above, individuals in modernity are enlisted by the state to exercise control over themselves.[99] Governmentality is partly achieved through expert, professional knowledge that represents particular perspectives and motivations.

Within the context of chemical deregulation, an example of this is the abundance of popular literature, shopping guides, and health promotion materials that have been published on the topic of green consumption, safe consumer selection, and nontoxic choices.[100] These primarily target pregnant women and parents of young children, with a focus on protecting the fragility of children's growing bodies from exposure to toxins.[101] These materials encourage participation in what MacKendrick calls "precautionary consumption," wherein the consumer examines food, household, or cosmetic product contents for synthetic chemicals in an effort to reduce exposure to toxins.[102] Attention is heavily directed toward all aspects of maternity, including the protection of pre-pregnancy maternal health.[103] As such, the process of such levels of self-monitoring, as well as the management of child health exposures, is labor-intensive.[104] What can reasonably be garnered from these institutions' emphasis on the individualization of risk and self-protection is that chemical exposure is an issue that can be mediated at the individual and family levels. The management of exposure to toxins is constructed as a caregiving responsibility that is traditionally defined as a role for women and mothers. There is a moral dimension to this, which we are regularly reminded of by discourses and norms that are part of our day-to-day practices, habits, and interactions. Moral discourses about good motherhood become internalized by individuals and influence our desire to meet the norms of "good mother," leading to self-surveillance. This illustrates a key theoretical insight from Foucault: conformity is achieved through desire.

It is now up to the individual to manage the individual's personal exposure to risk through monitoring and changing personal behavior. Mitchell Dean observes that technologies of agency—strategies rendering the individual actor responsible for his or her own actions—are paired with technologies of performance.[105] Self-monitoring is fostered through the commercial production of technologies of surveillance. Altering consumerist practices also conveys a sense of individual empowerment and agency through acts of "green" consumption.[106] Ultimately, this power also produces the types of bodies that society requires—disciplined bodies appropriate to the capitalist enterprise. The risk of chemical exposure is perceived as being manageable at the individual level, while simultaneously deflecting attention from states and industries' mismanagement of manufacture and distribution of chemicals.

Likewise, the public health emphasis on lifestyle factors and genes, rather than a focus on collective responsibility and institutional complicity, is a barrier to addressing cancer's environmental roots.[107] Public health organizations and agencies were formed 150 years ago to protect citizens from health threats. They were shaped by both the growth of scientific knowledge and the public acceptance of disease control as a public responsibility. While from the late nineteenth century through the mid-twentieth century public health organizations were concerned with public efforts to protect individuals, this promotion was accompanied by federal activities that promoted programs for individual health and values that supported social responsibility.[108] Today, political and ideological shifts within the government and across the country have shifted the perception of public health to a model that is based on a private market approach and led to a crisis in care and funding. U.S. public health organizations, including the American Cancer Society (ACS) and the CDC, emphasize self-protection but take a less active approach to the prevention of cancers linked to toxins and primarily focus on modifiable anthropogenic risk factors, such as nutrition, tobacco use, and excessive sun exposure. One reason for this is that factors such as these have yielded the most measurable results with regard to lowering cancer risk in the general population, and thus have resulted in successful policy and program interventions.[109] However, in distributing materials on contaminant avoidance, these institutions also minimize the role of larger social and political structures in contributing to environmental risk and their negative health consequences.[110] Suggestions are provided, for example, to reduce dioxin exposure by using fat-free or low-fat milk and using butter in moderation. To reduce arsenic risk, the National Institutes of Health recommends testing one's drinking water and eating a "well-balanced diet for good nutrition."[111]

These inconsistencies extend to health research and public health policies, where models often present individual responsibility and cultural explanations as organizing and theorizing principles. For example, the model of disease causation that dominates social epidemiological studies today, known as the "web of causation," draws attention to a number of interacting factors that might contribute to disease.[112] Although the inclusion of social factors is important for understanding health and illness, even researchers who use the web of causation model sometimes emphasize behavior and genes and downplay the role of social factors. Some researchers continue to subscribe to the notion of the individualization of risk, attributing responsibility for lifestyle and behaviors to the individual, as opposed to the larger social and environmental context.[113] Researchers often describe race as an "exposure," in the same way that one may be exposed to environmental conditions, such as radiation or environmental toxins. Demographic characteristics, such as gender and race, become further decontextualized within a "spiderless" web of causation, and the significance of these factors in determining health outcomes is distorted.[114] Despite numerous studies that link social variables to nonindividualized factors, the individualized model persists as the most dominant health discourse.

As a cultural ideology, individualism reinforces capitalist ideals of equal opportunity and the value of hard work. This works to the benefit of neoliberals who have sought to limit public expenditures to open new possibilities for private investment and protect private property, which is essential for the continual accumulation of capital. It stands in contrast to ideas about the "right" to health and justifies restrictions on rights to public services, saving businesses and the government money and shifting costs back to the consumer.

THE RISK SOCIETY

Approximately 608,570 Americans are expected to die of cancer in 2021, which translates to about 1,670 deaths per day.[115] About one in four Americans can expect a cancer diagnosis during their lifetime. Scientific literature provides substantial evidence of environmental causes of cancer that serve as a driving force in initiating tumor development and progression. Governments at all levels have a responsibility to strive to create the conditions in which people can be as healthy as possible, including identifying and preventing carcinogenic exposures. Yet, they currently fall short in providing structural support for communities living with environmental contamination.

Assaults on scientific integrity and science-based policy illustrate that there is much more to the concept of risk than simply probabilities and expected values. Many disasters are socially produced and result from human decision making. Through science, legal professions, and the media, industrial stakeholders will continue to influence definitions of risk while casting doubt on the scientific linkages between toxins and disease and shifting responsibility for the management of risk to individuals.[116]

German sociologist Ulrich Beck offers a useful framework for understanding the creation and management of hazards today. In his theory of the "risk society,"

Beck argues that contemporary society must deal with new types of risks that are self-created because of industrialization processes over which we have little control. They are distinguished from risks in what Beck terms "first modernity," an earlier phase of industrialized society during which disasters were predominantly naturally occurring and perceived of as fateful events. These disasters were largely managed by a bureaucratic state that assumed responsibility for structuring people's lives within the industrialized world. In turn, loyalty was given by the populace to the emerging institutions of modernity. Beck asserts that by the latter half of the twentieth century, the existing paradigm was challenged by the complexity of opportunity and risk associated with the spread of industrialization, resulting in risks and hazards unparalleled in human history. These "manufactured risks," which have the added detriment of having little historical reference, have emerged from advancements in science and technology. Beck argues that with technological and social changes since the 1960s, we are entering a "second modernity" characterized by the increasing occupation with debating, preventing, and managing risks that modern society has itself produced.[117]

According to Beck, risks are no longer confined by geographical or temporal boundaries, as they cross national lines and affect future generations. Issues such as climate change, the economy, terrorism, and nuclear threat illustrate the global commonality of risk. While risks in first modernity were managed (and manageable) by traditional institutions, such as the church, family, and the state, contemporary risk management is primarily under the jurisdiction of science, technology, and a market-driven economy. While scientific and industrial development plays a significant role in the creation of risks and hazards in the risk society, science has also become the primary institution for identifying and analyzing risks, and it operates with little transparency and poor accountability. Risk societies rely on a more complex system of production that requires specialization for management, policy development, and overall understanding and interpretation. The necessity for such specialized expertise leads to both purposeful and unintentional barriers to public access in acquiring environmental hazard information.

Because the production of risks is difficult to attach to an identifiable actor or institution, actors or institutions are not held accountable for the hazards generated by the risk society. Beck refers to this as "organized irresponsibility." Furthermore, it is increasingly unlikely that individuals harmed by the generated dangers can receive recourse due to the convoluted nature of source and accountability and the impossibility of calculating risk. Beck argues that a culture of fear emerges from the paradoxical fact that the institutions designed to control risk actually produce uncontrollability. He notes that "victims of hazards today are imperceptibly abandoned to the judgments, mistakes, and controversies of experts, and subjected to terrible psychological stresses." What is lost in the midst of the emphasis on scientific talk are the personal and social impacts on people's everyday lives.

It is not that Beck's theory rests with the conception of the world as an unsafe place to live. In the risk society, disproportionate amounts of risks lead to feelings of anxiety; to concern for safety and well-being.[118] As a consequence of weakened traditional institutions intended to safeguard public welfare and under the guise of democratic humanism, the powerful production of risks acts as a catalyst in changing public perceptions about the ability of state institutions to manage modern risks. Independent of institutions and empowered by knowledge, people are challenging the status quo and through social movements altering scientific and social institutions—a change Beck refers to as "subpolitics." Subpolitics, which involves forms of active citizenship, such as grassroots community action, has positive implications for both the environment and social justice, and its consequences may be as significant as traditional politics. For Beck, power is thus centered on the origin and diffusion of knowledge about risks.

Among other critiques of Beck's work over the years, this assumption—that social change is merely dependent on knowledge—ignores the cultural dimensions of rationality and reflection and the cultural embeddedness of social interaction. For example, as in the story of Clyde, I show that contamination stories are composed of anecdotal knowledge that residents share and to which residents have constant access. Yet, in spite of the federal EPA's discovery of PCBs at the former Whirlpool Park, the biggest conflict that emerged was among the residents themselves regarding what caused the cancer, rather than between the community and Whirlpool Corporation as the cause of contamination.

Understanding the broader context of neoliberalism and industrial influence on chemical regulation and risk assessment helps clarify how these systems contribute to the smokescreen of accountability. It is no surprise that subsequent community response to toxic exposure is often marked by conflict between residents, with science, albeit prone to obfuscation, being the definitive platform for most of these debates.

2 ▸ CANCER IN CLYDE AND "WILL-O'-THE-WISP THINGS"

Aℓℓᴇxᴀ ᴡᴀꜱ ᴇɪɢʜᴛ years old when she began experiencing head-aches, blurry and double vision, and dizziness. Her parents, Wendy and War-ren, thought she might be having eye problems and took her to the family doctor. After Alexa was unable to perform a straight-line walk, the doctor ordered an MRI. Alexa was diagnosed with medulloblastoma—a brain tumor—on May 11, 2006.

Around the time of her diagnosis, several new cancer cases occurred. In Feb-ruary 2006, twelve-year-old Tyler Hisey was diagnosed with acute myeloid leu-kemia (AML) and underwent seven months of chemotherapy at Saint Vincent's Hospital in Toledo (her younger brother would be diagnosed with acute lym-phoblastic leukemia two years later). Five-year-old Chase Berger had a thumb-sized malignant tumor called rhabdomyosarcoma removed from behind his eye in 2006. Kole Keller died of medulloblastoma two days before his sixth birthday in April 2007. Twenty-year-old Shilah Donnersbach died of Ewing's sarcoma in December of 2007.

As an increasing number of children in Clyde began being diagnosed with cancer, residents' curiosity and speculation grew. Although there did not seem to be a common denominator among the affected children, parents were noticing the prevalence of cancer diagnoses within their circles of acquaintances and within their own families. They recall that their initial reaction was not extremely dramatic. Rather, they thought it was "odd" that so many children were being diagnosed.

The school nurse was at the forefront of those noticing an increase in the occurrence of several different cancers, especially among elementary-age kids. Knowing that it was not typical for a small town to coincidentally have so many children with cancer at the same time, she was one of the first in the community to notify the local health department. In response to the increasing concerns from residents, the Sandusky County Department of Public Health (SCDPH) requested assistance from the Ohio Department of Health (ODH) in determining the incidence of childhood cancer among residents of Clyde City and Green Creek Township. The SCDPH also inquired if the incidence of cancer differed in a statistically significant way from that expected based on national cancer incidence rates.[1] Cancer cases were identified through the Ohio Cancer Incidence Surveillance System (OCISS).[2] Invasive cancers diagnosed from 1996 to 2006 were used in the analysis, and additional efforts were made to confirm that the data were as accurate and complete as possible, including contacting hospitals in Sandusky County to identify cancers not yet reported to the OCISS. The incidence of cancer among the study populations was compared with national cancer incidence rates from the Surveillance Epidemiology and End Results (SEER) Program of the National Cancer Institute.[3]

The agency's findings, released in the spring of 2007, indicated that a total of ten invasive cases of cancer were diagnosed from 1996 to 2006 among childhood residents of Clyde City and Green Creek Township. Males and females were affected equally, with the largest number being diagnosed in the fifteen-to-nineteen-years-of-age group. Brain and central nervous system cancers were the most diagnosed cancers. One case of each of the following cancers was also diagnosed: Ewing's sarcoma (soft tissue), Hodgkin's lymphoma, leukemia, osteosarcoma (bone), rhabdomyosarcoma, and testis. The number of cases observed was about twice the number expected, although this difference was not statistically significant at the 95 percent confidence interval. When expanding the study site to also include Riley, Townsend, and York Townships, however, the four-township region was determined to have a statistically significantly higher number of cancers than expected based on national comparison rates. Yet again, other than the cases of brain and other central nervous system cancer, no commonalities were found among the cases in the expanded scope of study. In contrast to the analyses for the eleven-year period, the ODH found statistically significantly higher-than-expected numbers of cancers for the five-year period of 2002–2006 for Clyde City and Green Creek Township, as well as the four-township population. Figure 3 shows the radius of the cancer cluster.

Even at the time of the ODH's health assessment, some affected families remember that although the problem of cancer was in the forefront of their

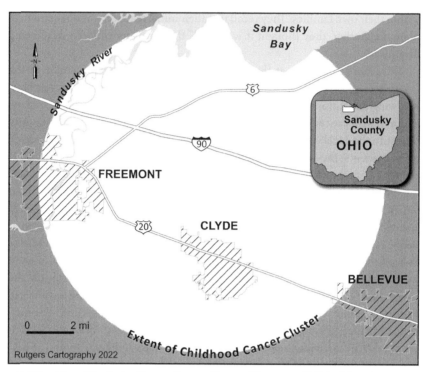

FIGURE 3. Map of Sandusky County Cancer Cluster. (Courtesy of Michael Siegal, Department of Geography, Rutgers University.)

minds, nobody was yet using the phrase "cancer cluster." Environmental toxins were also not initially discussed by health officials, and the community was slow to consider the possible role of toxins. However, there were exceptions within some families. A close friend to the Keller family, for instance, remembers that Kole Keller's doctors at Saint Jude Children's Research Hospital informed the family that what Kole had "was not something that was hereditary," and it was "very likely to have been caused by something environmental." During the ODH meeting when the results of the cancer incidence report were shared, families at the meeting expressed concerns about the possible role of environmental contamination and requested the involvement of the Ohio EPA and the ODH Bureau of Environmental Health.

In December 2008, the Sandusky County Combined General Health District (SCCGHD), the ODH Chronic Disease & Behavioral Epidemiological Section, the ODH Health Assessment Section (HAS), and the Ohio EPA Northwest District Office (NWDO) staff met with impacted families to discuss and address environmental concerns. The ODH discussed the five components of the completed exposure pathway, a measurement tool used by epidemiologists to identify how humans are exposed to chemicals in the environment, and how all five must be present to determine if the community's health was impacted. SCDPH staff conducted a case review of the Clyde City and Green Creek Township area for the years 1996–2006 using a standardized questionnaire developed by the ODH. The questionnaire gathered information concerning family history of cancer, parent/guardian work history, age of mom at conception, exposure to cigarette smoke and alcohol use, drinking water sources, school attendance, and other information in an attempt to identify factors that may have played a role in the development of these cancers. In February 2008, the case review was released to the public. Fourteen case families agreed to participate, but the exposure assessment did not reveal any common or individual factors that may have played a role in the childhood cancers.

Parents began to wonder if the commonalities between the cases were based on the histories of the parents, rather than the impacted children. The perceived thread that existed among the parents was loosely connected to their swimming at Whirlpool Park. Rumors were circulating that Whirlpool had dumped chemicals near the park, and that the company had pumped the pool full of water from the nearby creek, which might have been contaminated with chemicals.

Coinciding with the cancer cluster investigation, Whirlpool closed the park in 2006. It sold the property in 2008 to a family that planned to build a house on the property.

Alexa underwent surgery the day after her diagnosis, and a malignant tumor was removed. She developed delayed onset loss of speech, unsteadiness, and irritability—a syndrome known as cerebellar mutism—and underwent speech, physical, and occupational therapy. She underwent radiation therapy and nine cycles of chemotherapy, but the cancer returned in 2008. This time, it was treated with a combination of chemotherapy and stem cell therapy, the harvesting and transplant of which took place in Columbus, Ohio.

During the summer of 2008, ten-year-old Tanner Hisey was diagnosed with T-cell leukemia. Following the reports of Tanner's case and an additional child cancer case in the Clyde area over the 2008 summer months, renewed community concerns again centered on the environment as a likely cause—specifically the release of chemicals into air, land, and water from two nearby facilities, Whirlpool and the Vickery Environmental deep well injection waste disposal facility named after the nearby town of Vickery, Ohio.

The earliest documents related to wastewater in Ohio EPA files are dated 1973 and involve Whirlpool.[4] These files indicate that wastewaters from Whirlpool consisted of acidic tank wastewaters, acidic rinse waters, and floor and machinery washings. These wastewaters were treated using a lagoon system that involved treatment, clarification, and aeration prior to the wastewater being discharged to Raccoon Creek. Sludge was periodically removed from the primary lagoon and taken to a landfill. This continued for another sixteen years until 1989, when Whirlpool ceased the discharge of process wastewater to Raccoon Creek altogether and all wastewater effluent was diverted to the City of Clyde Wastewater Treatment Plant.

Vickery Environmental, Inc. (VEI) has run a regulated hazardous waste treatment, storage, and disposal facility since 1958. Throughout the 1960s, oil and industrial waste was pumped into surface impoundments. These are natural topographic depressions or human-made excavations that are designed to hold liquid wastes. The waste exceeded the capacity and created a storage issue, and by 1992 the impoundments were all closed. From 1976 to the present, hazardous waste has been injected into deep wells. Waste Management acquired the deep injection wells from Ohio Liquid Disposal, Inc., in 1978. There are seven wells drilled below the city's drinking water. Three wells were abandoned when they failed, meaning that the integrity of the well construction was compromised, making them not operational. Failed wells are a safety hazard in that they act as conduits for contaminants to move into deeper aquifers. In 1984, the Ohio attorney general filed a decree against Waste Management because of the threat to the environment. Four wells are still being operated to dispose of corrosives and acids, pickle liquor from iron and steel production, water from recycling operations, water from incinerator scrubbers and leachate recovered from other solid waste facilities. The total liquid waste disposed for all four wells in 2015 was 1.46 billion gallons.

Despite regulation of emissions from VEI by the EPA, red clouds of nitrogen dioxide, nitric oxide, and nitric gas have been visible from Clyde coming from VEI. Nitric oxide and nitric gas have also long been recognized as extremely toxic environmental pollutants. Nitrogen dioxide is easily absorbed through the lungs, and its inhalation can result in heart failure and sometimes death. In 2003, the EPA responded to a report but did not evacuate anyone. In 2006, the EPA reacted to another report and the fire department evacuated the area.

The Ohio EPA Emergency Response Unit has also dealt with two surface water releases with VEI—one in 1993 and the other in 2003. In both instances, a pipeline above ground failed. In 1993 alone, up to 800 gallons of waste acid flowed into Little Raccoon Creek, forming an orange residue. Surface water flowing onto the site was diverted by pumping the water to Little Raccoon Creek on the south side of Route 412, and the contaminated water and soil generated from the cleanup of the release were managed as hazardous waste.[5] In 2003, another pipeline broke, resulting in a release of waste acid that progressed to Meyers Ditch. The highest concentrations of hazardous waste found in the ditch were of lead, iron, nickel, and chromium, all of which cause risks for human health and the environment. Lead, for example, is stored in the bone but may affect any organ system. Overexposure can present as neurological symptoms in children and may cause high blood pressure and damage to the reproductive organs in adults. Overexposure to chromium may cause lung and respiratory tract cancer as well as kidney diseases. Some cases of overexposure to nickel have been associated with an increased risk of lung cancer. Roughly 71,000 gallons of contaminated storm water were collected and disposed of. Due to continuous rainfall, vacuum trucks could not keep up with the additional stormwater that was overwhelming the gate. Eventually, the main valve that emptied into Little Raccoon Creek had to be opened to prevent blowout. Samples determined that additional soil removal was necessary, but contaminated soil could not be removed until weather conditions in the area improved.

Using data from the EPA, residents' accounts, and old maps, Janice England—who founded an organization to provide information on open and closed dumpsites—identified six historical dump sites in the small town of Clyde, some of which pre-date Whirlpool's establishment in the town.[6] The Clyde Whirlpool plant has three dumps on its property that were left there from Clyde Porcelain Steel. Several other dumps and suspected dumps have been identified, including the Wickerham Drum site, the Whirlpool Manufacturing site, and the Golembioski dump. Based on residents' accounts and previous ownership, dump sites were also suspected at Cherry Street Park, near Clyde High School, and near McPherson Cemetery. Additionally, although not listed on the EPA's National Priorities List, the property at the former Clyde Paint & Supply Co., Inc., is currently registered as an active Superfund site—an area designated by the EPA as a polluted location requiring long-term response to cleanup of hazardous material due to the contamination of soil with xylene. Exposure to xylene can occur via inhalation, ingestion, or eye or skin contact and causes health effects from both acute and chronic exposure. The main effect of xylene exposure is depression of the central nervous system. For a small town, this is a notable number of dump sites that reflects a national trend of industries that follow the path of least resistance when deciding where to locate hazardous waste sites and other polluting facilities. Several decades of research show that minority and low-income neighborhoods and communities are disproportionately targeted by industries because they have fewer resources and political clout to oppose the siting of unwanted facilities.[7]

The Ohio EPA had also responded to one significant disaster from Whirlpool's Clyde facility in 2003 when 2,700 gallons of porcelain mixed with water were "accidentally" released into a storm sewer that discharged into Raccoon Creek. Porcelain enameling activities are common in major household appliance manufacturing, and because of the amount of toxic metals present, the sludges generated during wastewater treatment typically contain substantial amounts of toxic metals.[8]

Whirlpool took responsibility for the cleanup, and there was no reported significant damage to the creek or environment.[9] The Toxics Release Inventory (TRI) Program indicates that the company has otherwise operated in compliance with the EPA's environmental regulations.[10]

Despite the families' concern, the topic of the environment remained peripheral to the concerns of the ODH. Alexa's mother, Wendy, recalls that around the year 2008, the director of the ODH, Robert Indian, informed the affected families that "there was nothing more he could do, and it would be up to them to ask the EPA for assistance." Wendy remembers thinking, "By the time they got involved, it was like . . . you've got to be kidding. This was something that he should have talked about. It should have been brought up then so that they could have started checking environmentally right away, but I mean it was like two years later."

Finally, in January 2009, the Ohio EPA began monitoring both short- and long-term air quality samples throughout the area. They found no elevated levels of pollutants that would indicate a public health concern, including volatile organic compounds (VOCs) or heavy metals.[11] The agency also evaluated drinking water quality from public water systems (City of Clyde and Northern Ohio Rural Water) and six private wells used by residents with impacted children. However, while a few naturally occurring substances were identified at elevated concentrations in the water well samples, those that exceeded a U.S. EPA health advisory level or secondary maximum contaminant level did not have carcinogenic health implications.[12] The Ohio EPA also inspected eight local industries' compliance with environmental laws, but again, no environmental risk related to a cancer-causing agent or condition was identified. Also in January 2009, the Ohio Department of Health Bureau of Environmental Health Indoor Environments Section met with SCCGHD and reviewed inspection reports for the period 1990–2008 of six area schools, but no significant environmental quality or safety issues were identified. A later report would rule out the possibility of radiation at the schools, along with other locations in the area.[13] The Ohio EPA would also rule out the possibility of toxic chemicals at levels of public health concern in tested soils in the area.[14]

By the spring of 2009, Alexa Brown had lost the use of her legs and the cancer had worsened in her spine. Her parents took her to a hospital in Vermont with hopes of having Alexa participate in an experimental trial. The new trial required that participants not receive chemotherapy for at least three weeks. During that time, cancer cells attacked Alexa's body, and she was sent home because the MRI results disqualified her. The MRI showed that the cancer in her spine had grown and also returned in her brain. She was put on an aggressive nutritional supplement plan. On July 3, 2009 Alexa had an excruciatingly painful headache and was taken to the hospital. In the middle of the night, she became unable to communicate. She was sent home with hospice care, where her family had one final month to spend with her. Alexa's father Warren remembers spending late nights sitting on their front porch. As Alexa got closer to the end, no one in the house slept and they were with Alexa all the time. Eleven-year-old Alexa died on Thursday, August 6, 2009.

The regular course of life that most people take for granted would forever be altered for the Brown family. They met and received support from Ohio senator Sherrod Brown, who became an advocate for them in their search for federal attention to the issue. In November of that year, Senator Sherrod Brown's office contacted the Centers for Disease Control and Prevention (CDC) to request its involvement in the Clyde cancer investigation, but after reviewing ODH's cancer investigation efforts, representatives from the CDC responded stating that the ODH investigation was comprehensive and exhaustive and that no further action was warranted by their agency. In February 2011, Senator Sherrod Brown sent another letter to the CDC, as well as to U.S. EPA administrator Lisa Jackson's office, requesting increased involvement from the federal agencies in the Clyde cancer investigation. Again, the CDC responded by calling the efforts of the supporting agencies "comprehensive and exhaustive."

It was not until five years after the ODH became involved in studying the cancer cluster that a supplemental questionnaire was developed and administered to include additional questions about the possible role of environmental toxins. In May 2011, a decision was made to expand the 2007 case review to thirty-five cases in the area because the ODH found consistencies among the types of cancers and victim profiles in the original study of twenty cases. They broadened the geographical boundaries to account for a possibly wider affected area and in hopes they would be able to gather more information.

The affected families were not convinced by the "exhaustive and comprehensive" environmental review. In the words of Alexa's father, Warren, they felt that the EPA and Ohio Department of Health investigations were "underfunded, undermanned, and possibly performed by those who don't have quite the skill set that those on the federal level maintain." They were skeptical that representatives from the Ohio Health Department and other representatives from the Ohio EPA would not follow through and, because the agencies were slow to get the study going, there was a feeling that perhaps they missed an opportunity to detect toxins earlier. Warren explained, "Therein lies part of my skepticism with the whole system—why should a family, why should someone have to be approached by an attorney to start conducting tests that we've asked to have conducted years and years and years ago? . . . Their activities have been met with skepticism in my eye, they've been met also and it seems somewhat juxtaposed because there's also a level of appreciation. At least they did come and try to do something, but they just didn't do enough."

Investigative reporter Scott Taylor from Cleveland's 19 Action News questioned then federal EPA director Lisa Jackson in June 2011 as she toured the headquarters of the Moen faucet manufacturing corporation about one hour east of Clyde in North Olmsted, Ohio. He asked her when the federal EPA would meet with parents in Clyde, but she stated that she was not aware of the Clyde cancer cluster. The EPA later sent a statement to 19 Action News stating that Lisa

Jackson and her senior regional staff would "meet with the residents of Clyde, and will fulfill that commitment."[15] However, Jackson never fulfilled that promise, adding to residents' sense of disillusionment with the lack of follow-through and governmental intervention. A recurring feeling that residents expressed was a need for reassurance that this issue would be taken care of. Contributing to the sense of betrayal some felt by the government, residents were also frustrated by the length of time the situation had remained unresolved, and that the response to the problem was not strong and immediate. In the words of one resident, Marilyn, "Who's helping these people?! They can't get no answers, they can't get no answers! That's what makes me angry, that's when I say, why is not, why isn't anyone gonna help the children? Who's gonna protect the children if we don't?!"

In 2012, Robert Indian, chief of the state's comprehensive cancer-control program at ODH, announced that the department would take a "very twenty-first-century" approach to cancer—one that involved avoiding time spent on cancer cluster cases whenever possible and spending more time boosting prevention and early detection of disease. "There's more payoff in that, and it does more good than continuing to pursue these will-o'-the-wisp things," he said. Cancer cluster investigations "use a lot of resources, raise expectations, and you find nothing."[16] Indian's comments conveyed a defeatist, passive attitude that was disconcerting to the families in Clyde fighting to find answers on behalf of their children. From Alexa's mother's perspective, it meant "We don't wanna find out."

General lack of enthusiasm when it comes to government intervention in addressing or correcting environmental contamination is both confounding and contradictory in that the very agencies dedicated to the task of assessment and remediation appear reluctant to engage. Despite Indian's political-speak characterization of their response being a twenty-first-century approach, this response was not part of a broader change in the way cancer was researched across the country. Although his chosen words were insensitive, former Ohio Department of Health director Robert Indian's statement about disease clusters as "will-o'-the-wisp things" was likely conflated with the limitations of the current systems for effective risk assessment.

A combination of factors contributes to what might be perceived as a letdown by the very offices designated to protect the public from such disasters. Lax regulation of the chemical industry has created potential hazards that experts are incapable of managing, let alone identifying. Whereas the impact of prevention and early detection initiatives can be measured, it is notoriously difficult to link a single cause to a cluster of cancer clusters. When Indian redirected the focus of his health agency to encouraging preventive measures among the populace, he was confronting the fact that his agency in all probability did not have the capacity to fix problems such as disease clusters.

All levels of government are also pro-industry to some degree. At the state and federal levels, both government and industry-based businesses have incen-

tives to avoid massive financial loss that would incur in terms of cleanup and liability. Local governments tend to also favor industry because of the revenue and
jobs industry produces. Many towns offer tax incentives to companies because
the town benefits through taxing plant workers. It was reported that the Whirlpool plant in Benton Harbor had more than $550 million in stockpiled business
tax credits that could be used to offset its future income or taxes and could also
be carried over year to year for the next twenty years.[17] In 2018, the city finance
director for Clyde observed that roughly two-thirds of Clyde's budget came
from taxes paid by Whirlpool, its workers, suppliers, and vendors. It is not surprising that a pro-industry government would be an unwilling participant in an
environmental debate that it was not only incapable of solving—either politically or scientifically—but also incentivized to keep the water muddy. Consequently, the responsibility for protection was turned back onto the community
of Clyde itself.

Though not included in the public health assessments, in addition to children
many adults in the communities of Clyde and Green Springs have also been
affected by illness and disease and have presented with an inordinate number of
unusual and multiple cancers, including spine cancer, eye tumors, and cancer
of the spleen.[18] Betty, a sixty-nine-year-old resident of Clyde, recalls coming to
this realization with her husband when she was being treated for her cancer: "We
started looking around saying, 'Jeez it's not just the kids—it's the adults.' And
I started taking chemo and everything down here at North Coast. There were a
lot of people. People I knew, you know, 'What are you doing in here? Why are
you in here?' 'Well, I have cancer.' 'Yeah, I do too.'"

In February 2012, six years after the initial involvement of the ODH and Ohio
EPA, the U.S. EPA finally became involved. There was a perception among some
affected families that, whether an issue of territoriality or competency, the Ohio
EPA took offense to their request for U.S. EPA involvement. Nevertheless, the
U.S. EPA stepped in and conducted an assessment of fourteen dump sites identified by the Ohio EPA and Clyde residents but did not discover contaminants
that warranted removal.[19] During the initial investigation of these sites, the EPA
established a telephone hotline to elicit information from local residents regarding additional potential dump sites in the area. The EPA received approximately
ninety anonymous calls to the hotline, with enough information to warrant site
assessments at three additional locations.

Those families questioned government agencies' resistance to testing all sites
for possible contamination, expressing frustration that nobody was taking them
seriously. "We can't test every dump site that people tell us about," the on-scene
coordinator for the EPA told one resident who was worried about a dumping
ground next to Whirlpool Park. One family recounted instances where they
attempted to contact state-level politicians, including Governor John Kasich,
but received no response. Governor Kasich expressed concern around election

time, even requesting to talk to the family's ill son on the phone, but stopped short when it came to doing anything meaningful. Others felt that had the contamination been validated by the ODH or EPA representatives, then perhaps skeptical members of the community would view the concerned residents' complaints as more legitimate. Complex, conflicting, and delayed distribution of information from government agencies added to residents' frustration with their lack of recourse.

Eyewitness accounts of illegal dumping and rumors of reprisal directed at whistleblowers added to the conflict that erupted between residents regarding the causes of the cancer. Stories circulated involving eyewitness accounts of the corporation appropriating the community's natural resources and using them as distribution points for waste without consent. Accounts of dumping in the creek, Whirlpool Park, and sites west of town were accepted as common knowledge by many. Josephine, a four-time cancer survivor who had previously lived near Whirlpool Park and was part of the lawsuit, had her well tested for toxins with the help of her attorney because the health department had previously skipped testing for her well. "They never came to my house," she explained, "but I know that they tested. . . . They did a whole bunch of testing over at Whirlpool Park. Right after they did that, boom—the park was closed."

Her attorney informed her that there were fifteen cancer-causing chemicals in her water. She remembers seeing Whirlpool employees dump at the park:

> It was usually on the closing day—they were closed on Mondays. It wasn't every Monday, but it was often . . . and they would bring a big dump truck and they would open up the gates, back it into this little area and dump this garbage— canisters, barrels, sometimes cement, buckets. I never did photograph the trucks. I wasn't out to get anybody—I've never been that kind of a person. I did call the EPA, and they never got back to me. And that water that filled the pool came outta the creek. So that stuff that they were dumpin' in that pile went into the creek and then went into a slight filtration system they had and that water went right into the swimming pool all those years. It was a mess down there.

After the filing of the lawsuit, concerns were also expressed that the Whirlpool factory was releasing toxic fumes at night because of a noxious odor detected near the plant after dark. A potent burning chemical/plastic odor that permeated the air and the "Whirlpool smell" at night became a talking point at public meetings. Observers stated that the smell went away shortly after the filing of the lawsuit. Suspicions were also shared about occupational hazards within the Whirlpool facility itself. Carl, a former Whirlpool employee who suffered from heart problems and Parkinson's disease, questioned whether his heart problems were related to his thirty-six years in management at Whirlpool:

I worked in finishes. We worked with a lot of hazardous chemicals in that area, but when we first put in a powder coat system, at that time, we didn't know when we first put it in, but the makeup of that powder coat had a known carcinogen in it and could form mutations. And I, we did lose some operators with heart issues from there. . . . We've had some cancer in the area where they had a lot of oil mess, but you know, I think that that doesn't, to me, that's not any different than any other manufacturing plant that has the hazardous chemicals or has the oil misting process. I think it's just the nature of the work, so I guess that's kinda . . . I don't like to say that it's definitely Whirlpool. But yeah we have had deaths that I've questioned whether, I thought probably came from the work conditions.

Erika, who had worked for Whirlpool for thirty-seven years, expressed her early suspicion that the working environment there might be making employees sick:

I had always heard rumors at work that Whirlpool dumped in the creek out there just to get rid of stuff without having to pay to have it hauled away. I heard it from guys who were told to do it. And then when I was about six, my dad and I would go mushroom huntin' just west of town right outside the city limits. There used to be an apple orchard and back in one corner there was a bunch of old barrels. They were green, with different colored stuff coming out of 'em, and my dad would say, "Don't go back there." It was one of [Whirlpool's] dumping grounds and my dad was employed at Whirlpool for probably forty years. So I remember from back then, him saying that stuff was there. And then there was that place on Main Street that a friend of mine grew up in, and my dad said Whirlpool had buried barrels in their front yard.

Residents began to wonder at what point those actions occurred and under what authority those liberties were assumed. One noted that the illegality of the acts had to be known or else the dumping would not have been of such a surreptitious nature.

Upon receiving tips to the anonymous hotline, the U.S. EPA found contaminants at a residential property on the west side of Clyde, which included semivolatile organic compounds (SVOCs), Target Analyte List (TAL) metals, and Toxicity Characteristic Leaching Procedure (TCLP) metals.[20] These chemicals and heavy metals are of great concern as soil pollutants because they can threaten the health of people and animals through the food chain. A number of contaminants were found at the former Clyde Paint and Supply Co. site that exceeded the applicable screening criterion, including a number of VOCs, SVOCs, TAL metals, and polychlorinated biphenyls (PCBs). In addition, the hotline tips included information that Whirlpool had filled in the area surrounding and under the basketball court in the former Whirlpool Park site with a black sludge-like material.[21] In September 2012, the federal agency completed six soil borings at the former Whirlpool Park site. Results found PCBs present at levels that exceeded U.S. EPA Regional Screening Levels for residential properties. PCBs detected around the basketball court ranged from two to nine feet thick. In addition, the metals cobalt and nickel were also identified at levels that exceeded the EPA's screening criterion.[22] In public statements, Whirlpool denied knowledge of the polluted soil at Whirlpool Park, although plaintiffs had identified drawings on file in the Sandusky County courthouse that showed that the basketball court, tennis court, and pool were built after Whirlpool bought the park.

The EPA uses national and regional policies, as well as site-specific considerations like community interest, to guide when and to what extent community engagement may be appropriate for each PCB cleanup, storage, and disposal approval that the agency issues. Despite the community concern about the PCBs, the U.S. EPA did not notify residents about the discovery of the toxic sludge at the former Whirlpool Park site. Rather, members of the community discovered the report online in November 2012. Karen, who lives near the site, expressed frustration that the EPA did not adequately inform local residents of the nearby danger of toxins at the time of the house visits the EPA had made over the summer. To residents, withholding that information felt dishonest and disrespectful. Karen stated,

> The EPA came and sat at our table and they asked us if we witnessed any kind of dumping and trucks. They asked us, you know, what kind of illness that we had. At the time they came here they knew exactly what was found over there. I can't believe that they do not tell the immediate people within the . . . at least I mean when I looked up the hazards, cautions, and cleanup, it said it went out like maybe 1,500 feet, maybe 2,000 feet that they would evacuate people or have people not be drinking their water, you know, boil. And I'm thinking we are all right here and they're disturbing soil that they already know has PCBs. It's like they don't give us the courtesy and consideration.

Concerned residents had no choice but to become their own advocates to locate information about PCBs. Through social media, a network developed among concerned residents. Members also began educating themselves about toxins through online resources. Although the EPA had discovered PCBs in the spring, its report was not made available until the fall and it did not notify residents— even those who lived near the site. Michelle, who lived in close proximity to Whirlpool Park, remembered learning about the EPA report from a friend on Facebook:

> I went on the Internet and looked up PCBs and exactly what they're from and what they can cause. My main concern was my well water because my well is right

in front of the house here. When I found out that the PCB sludge was nine feet thick, I was really concerned about that living out here. And I had two dogs that died. We lost Bear that spring, and he was age five. Then last year we lost Max around the same time, and he was age six. They should live longer than that. The only thing we gave them other than dog food was water.

To add to locals' frustration, residents were never notified about cleanup efforts, and there were concerns that disrupting the PCB-laced soil would put them at a greater risk of toxin exposure. They wanted to be given a choice to leave their homes at the time of cleanup. Adding to the confusion, the EPA did not provide residents with the agency's contact information at the time of the house visits. When some residents finally made phone contact with the EPA in an attempt to clarify these unanswered questions about the cleanup, they were sidelined by a string of transfers, disconnections, and recorded responses.

Residents expressed frustration not only with the quality of Ohio EPA, ODH, and U.S. EPA investigations but also with the promptness of their response from the local to state to federal level. Alexa Brown's father remembers having an early suspicion that the agencies' efforts would not materialize:

I was reading a document today that was produced from the public meeting we held in 2008 at the Clyde high school. Alexa accompanied us to this meeting. And I sat there and I can remember hearing Robert Indian and others from Ohio EPA and Ohio Department of Health speak, and I recall distinctly thinking how skeptical I was. You know I just, you know you're saying all the right words, but are you really gonna follow through on what you're doing, do you really actually even know what you're doing? . . . I was encouraged when the U.S. EPA came in because they seem to have a much higher level of skills and they were bringing equipment that was far more technical to what Ohio EPA had. But again, the luster they had in my eyes at that point in time has become very lack luster now because they've not stayed the task. . . . They just didn't do enough.

Ultimately, impacted families turned to the legal system and to alternative sources of scientific proof in their pursuit of identifying who was responsible and who would be held accountable. The park's current owners, who had planned to build a home on the land until they learned about the toxins there, filed a lawsuit against the company alleging that Whirlpool misrepresented the condition of the park and did not disclose the contamination. Frustrated with the slow progress being made, affected families hired Alan Mortensen, a Utah-based personal injury attorney with ties to the area, along with Toledo-based firm Charles E. Boyk Law Offices, LLC, for legal help with their search for answers. When Mortensen became involved, the families had a renewed sense of hope for resolution as the lawyers and their team of scientists conducted independent environmental tests on their behalf. One of the tests performed involved testing the air and dust in the attics of affected families' homes. This was a test that families had requested from the Ohio EPA years earlier but were denied. While the team of lawyers and scientists were expecting to find evidence of PCBs in the dust, since PCBs (among other hazardous chemicals) were discovered at Whirlpool Park, the environmental tests revealed high levels of benzaldehyde instead. The levels of benzaldehyde indicated to the scientists that other chemicals may have once been present in the homes. In a sense, they interpreted benzaldehyde as a marker chemical—perhaps a remnant of two other chemicals that had burned and vaporized. With these findings, a class action lawsuit was filed against Whirlpool Corporation, citing, in part, the use of benzaldehyde in its manufacturing process. The lawsuit claimed that when Whirlpool ran out of places to dump sludge, the company resorted to burning the waste, causing the residual benzaldehyde to "blanket the entire Clyde area."[23] The lawsuit also claimed that benzaldehyde and other toxins were responsible for illness among the plaintiffs.

A study by W. M. Kluwe, C. A. Montgomery, H. D. Giles, and J. D. Prejeau revealed negative health effects of exposure to benzaldehyde in rats and mice, but studies within the toxicology literature remain sparse.[24] For this reason, benzaldehyde has not undergone a complete evaluation and determination under the U.S. EPA's Integrated Risk Information System (IRIS) program for evidence of human carcinogenic potential.[25] In contrast, and characteristic of the "innocent until proven guilty" regulatory system, the U.S. FDA has stated that the substance is "generally regarded as safe."[26]

The day after the lawyers and their team released their benzaldehyde findings, the Ohio Department of Health released an informational sheet stating that the chemical is nontoxic and commonly found in food and household items. Graphics on the flyer included colorful gumballs, ripe cherries, a bountiful harvest of fruit, a tray of baked goods, and a cup of frozen yogurt—innocuous illustrations of Americana. The types of graphics on the fact sheet are not an out-of-the-ordinary model for fact sheets that the Ohio Department of Health has released in the past. But one might speculate as to the timing of the release of the informational sheet, which was quickly and widely distributed. It was published in the local newspaper, and according to one interviewee, was even handed out at the building where residents pay utility bills. The families were irked by the ODH's flyer and expressed concern that this was an attempt to undermine their work. Some felt that although it was the Health Department that led the community to believe that illness was likely linked to environmental toxins, it was now backpedaling on the issue.

Whirlpool was quick to suppress concerns at the plant by distributing pamphlets that reiterated the ODH assertion regarding the safety of benzaldehyde. In addition to public statements clearing themselves of responsibility, the company sent employees home with a paper that made it clear that they would "vigorously defend our company, our community, and our employees."

However, after the Agency for Toxic Substances and Disease Registry (ATSDR) reviewed the indoor dust sampling conducted by the scientists at the request of the U.S. EPA, ATSDR identified factual inaccuracies. They determined that all the benzaldehyde levels were accidentally calculated incorrectly and were actually at levels below the EPA Preliminary Remediation Goals (PRGs).[27]

Meanwhile, under the supervision of the U.S. EPA, Whirlpool Corporation was given the authority to conduct its own site assessment of Whirlpool Park using AECOM, an outside contractor with roots in the manufacturing and chemical distribution industry. EPA's contractors, Weston Solutions, Inc. (Weston), provided oversight during the site assessment conducted by Whirlpool. The EPA collected a subset of split samples during the site assessment that was equal to about 5 percent of the total samples collected by AECOM.[28] In addition to EPA oversight with Weston, HzW Environmental Consultants, LLC, represented the current property owner and collected split samples during the site assessment. The site assessment activities focused on identifying potential sources of soil and water contamination.[29] After reviewing the findings submitted by Whirlpool's contractor, the U.S. EPA determined that the sampling activities were conducted in accordance with the approved guidelines. In line with AECOM's findings, the U.S. EPA determined that PCBs were the only contaminants of concern found to be above regulatory standards.[30] Removal of PCB-contaminated waste was set to be regulated for cleanup and disposal in accordance with the EPA's protocols for the management of PCB waste.

Some felt that Whirlpool spokesman Jeff Noel downplayed the presence of PCBs when he stated that "it's not uncommon to find these items in what is clearly fill material, fill dirt."[31] The assessment conducted by Whirlpool acknowledged that some of the improvements they made to the property, including the installation of the tennis and basketball courts, involved importing fill dirt into the park. The company denied responsibility for the dumping and released the following statement to the public: "In conclusion, the site assessment found no health risk and no evidence of hazardous illegal dumping. Using the site assessment as a scientific basis, Whirlpool will now work with the U.S. EPA and the OEPA on the development and implementation of an appropriate remediation plan."[32]

The statement revealed an attempt to conflate science with two unsubstantiated claims that the study found "no health risk and no evidence of hazardous illegal dumping." The company claimed that the site was safe but did not have any evidence to support their claim. While refusing to allow victims to have the sites in question independently tested, Whirlpool's representative, the vice president of communications and public affairs, was careful not to alienate the community. He explained, "We understand where the families are coming from. We have great empathy for the families. Our issue is with attorneys who have used no science, no fact."[33]

Prior to the federal EPA ban of PCBs in the late 1970s, the oily substance was used as a dielectric fluid in capacitors of large appliances to regulate electricity flow. The EPA mandates that any material containing more than fifty parts per million of PCBs be placed in a chemical landfill. In 2020, there were approximately forty PCB disposal facilities and fifty commercial storage facilities across the country, but only ten chemical landfills were established in the ten years after the PCB ban. It is plausible that the cost of transporting and dumping the PCB sludge would have been a deterrent for the appliance manufacturers to comply with EPA rules.

The PCB sludge was finally removed from the former Whirlpool Park property in 2016. The park exists now as a large, excavated lot.

When nonpublic courses of actions, such as the improper dumping of toxic waste or other methods of contamination, are imposed upon a community without the community's knowledge or consent, trust is replaced with suspicion and the contract between the community and industry corrodes. But the issues in Clyde also initiated a cycle of mistrust between affected families and the government agencies involved. The families, feeling as if they were being intentionally misdirected, expressed doubt in public officials' actual knowledge and abilities to address their problems and questioned the truthfulness of the EPA and Whirlpool's findings. Some suspected that the EPA and ODH were not aggressively investigating the cause of illness because Whirlpool was "paying them off." For many others in Clyde, there was also still a general expectation that the state would step in and fix the problem. Although the fundamental beliefs about how the government is supposed to work seem to have been shaken by the cancer cluster issue, some residents still held onto the perception that the government protects its citizens. Josephine explained, "You gotta trust 'em, you know? We can't do anything about it. What do we know?"

In spite of the federal EPA's discovery of PCBs at the former Whirlpool Park, a major conflict emerged among the residents themselves regarding what caused the cancer, rather than between the community and Whirlpool Corporation as the cause of contamination. Most areas of contention related to the debate surrounding what constitutes legitimate knowledge. This community split ultimately benefited the Whirlpool Corporation by contributing to a lack of cohesive demand for accountability, leading frustrated victims to sue the company. While theories and accusations were circulating throughout the town, the lawsuit further divided the community into different camps, with most residents in support of Whirlpool or choosing to remain uninvolved in the issue, a point illustrated by the poor turnout at public meetings concerning the cancer cluster. Many residents chose to not inform themselves about the issue, indicating a resistance to wanting to know about the problem in the first place.

Some plaintiffs felt certain that, given the large number of calls to the EPA tip line, with information surfacing about dumping in the community, someone would surely come forward to help their case. But this did not happen. Keith, a fifty-five-year-old press operator at Whirlpool, met with a former laborer inside the plant who disclosed to him questionable practices regarding the disposal of waste. When asked if she intended to become involved, the laborer declined, saying, "I don't want any part to do with talking." Another former employee of Whirlpool was enthusiastic about helping the lawyers expose the potential liability of the company but ultimately backed out.

Residents skeptical of the environmental/toxin link were confounded by the lack of a common denominator among the cancer cases. Specifically, they wondered why certain family members in the same household who were exposed to the same air, water, and other environmental factors got cancer, while other members of the household did not. Others stated that they would be more concerned about chemical contamination and pollution from Whirlpool if only they had "scientific proof." In Julie's words, "How are we compared to everywhere else? I haven't seen, we haven't become real involved I guess with, um, absolute facts."

Complicating the issue were implications that, if there were chemicals in Clyde, they were likely legacy chemicals from prior agricultural and industrial sources. After the filing of the lawsuit, a longtime resident submitted an article to the widely circulated local paper, the *Clyde Enterprise*, which directed the community's attention to the hazardous spray used in the past on the fruit farms on the outskirts of town in the past. And although there was substantial evidence for further investigation of Whirlpool as a possible source of contamination in the face of the PCB discovery at Whirlpool Park, some residents were not even convinced that Whirlpool was responsible for the PCB sludge buried there. One woman speculated that perhaps another company from out of town trespassed onto the property and dumped the contaminants there without Whirlpool's knowledge. Another explanation was the suspicion that trains traveling from the south may be dispersing toxins throughout the community via the wind. And when asked how elevated rates of cancer in such a small area could be explained, most on the side of Whirlpool explained this as a matter of genes and individual lifestyle.

Defeatism associated with the improbability of resolution created a sense of, "How can you worry when it's out of your control?" Some residents discounted evidence of a mass occurrence of cancer by generalizing the disease as inevitable and something that would occur anyway. The prevalence of illness at the Whirlpool facility itself, as described by many employees and others, was considered by some to be an expected occupational hazard. Fatalistic comments such as "the damage to my health has already been done" seemed to camouflage residents' anxiety about having an illness, about Whirlpool leaving, their losing jobs, and the changing identity of the town.

Fifty-year-old Shelby explained: "My faith is, if I'm, if I'm supposed to have cancer, I'm going to get it. If I'm not supposed to, I won't." Others minimized the significance of the disease cluster by asserting that it is not unique to Clyde and that one's life is predetermined by God. In Julie's words, "Other places have hurricanes, and more tornadoes than we have, and so there are other forms of problems. God's kinda got a plan for you and it's gonna get you no matter where you're at." Similarly, Barb likened the disease cluster to that of the natural phenomenon of tornadoes in Oklahoma: "It's kinda like the Oklahoma people. We're coming out of our storm shelters, and well, you know, we're Oklahomans—what can you do? We're gonna stay here. I mean, what are you gonna do?"

The assumption that "you can't fight city hall" contributed to a sense of non-confrontational inaction. There was also speculation that some residents simply did not care enough about the issue, or that they would pay more attention to the issue if they were personally affected. Remaining neutral was a way of taking a side without inviting unwanted attention, and doing nothing had its own implication of passive action. Ultimately, decisions such as these made by residents to remain uninvolved worked to the benefit of those suspected of generating the contamination.

CONCLUSION

The Centers for Disease Control and Prevention (CDC), the National Cancer Institute (NCI), and the EPA assist states with investigating disease clusters. Each year, state and local health departments respond to more than 1,000 inquiries about suspected cancer clusters, with most being determined to not be cancer clusters through the process of telephone interviewing.[34] When health officials do investigate a suspected disease cluster community, it is usually the result of political pressure, public attention, and/or the media, as was the case with Clyde.[35]

The slow response from the local, state, and federal government to investigate the cause of disease in Clyde reflects a political resistance common to other disease cluster cases, the most infamous example being Love Canal, New York. What we learned from the case of Love Canal was that it was not an environmental accident. Rather, it was a case of flagrant corporate negligence. For ten years, this residential neighborhood was used as a toxic chemical waste dump by Hooker Electrochemical Company, which then sold the canal to the Niagara Falls School Board for one dollar, and a new elementary school was built. Rather than addressing the actual problems related to citizens' health, the legal system ignored scientific evidence and conveniently favored corporate interests.[36] This instance became an example of how risk assessment, amplified in part by the limited resources allotted to operate regulatory systems, allowed industrial financial concerns to override challenges evinced by environmental harm.

In 2011, some U.S. senators, including Ohio's Democratic senator Sherrod Brown, began pushing for a federal law that would strengthen protection requirements for children and communities from disease clusters, in part by increasing federal funding toward such investigations.[37] A bill to direct the administrator of the Environmental Protection Agency to investigate and address cancer and disease clusters, including in infants and children, was introduced to Congress but has never been enacted. Because of the wealth of toxicology literature demonstrating harmful human health effects, environmental groups such as the Natural Resources Defense Council believe that toxic chemicals are likely to be responsible for the dozens of disease clusters identified across the United States and therefore should be better regulated. Republicans on congressional environmental committees, however, have expressed an ideological position emerging from neoliberalism and post-truth—concerns about over-regulation by the EPA, especially with a lack of scientific proof.[38]

The community of Clyde faced institutional barriers that inhibited growth of equitable forms of risk governance and the political agency of citizens. As with residents in other contaminated communities, families were forced to become their own advocates. Some turned to the literature on toxins to self-educate. One family even reached out to well-known environmental whistleblower Erin Brockovich for help. When the plaintiffs felt that they had exhausted all other options, they turned to attorneys and experts to take the lead in the search for answers. Paradoxically, residents increasingly became dependent on science and experts in their efforts to find justice and resolution. The willingness to challenge Whirlpool and stand up against the unassailable science, albeit with their own experts, was driven in part by a questioning in the effectiveness of modern governmental health and environmental agencies. These acts of self-agency were hampered when even the plaintiffs' team of "experts" lost their ability to provide certainty. The eventual withdrawal of the lawsuit further illustrates the difficulties of seeking resolution for toxic contamination when legal decisions regarding causes of illness must be based on evidence that is difficult to produce.

One insight that we can draw from the failures of government and industry is that neither can adequately address community contamination and its impacts on health. The lack of inclusion of cancer-stricken adults in the public health assessments highlights a diminished scrutiny within the U.S. regulatory system and encourages limits on resources directed to research, tracking, and prevention of toxic exposures. Families in Clyde searching for answers were keenly aware of these weaknesses. They questioned why health agencies were only searching for known causes of illness when there might be other existing chemicals or combinations therein that had not yet been linked to cancer. Some implicitly identified the limitations of health-tracking data as related to the current status of illnesses within the community, noting that several new cases of child-hood cancer since the 2006 assessment were not reflected in the statistics. Even prior to the initial involvement of the health departments and EPA, residents experienced a sense of defeat, with some resigning to the inevitability that this problem would be unsolvable.

The burgeoning mutual interdependence of industry and government help determine risk exposure. Lack of institutional accountability foreshadows a lack of community consensus about the problem of contamination or its solutions. Considered as a whole, although the narratives contain contradictions, conflicting viewpoints depict Clyde as a risk community whose residents were grappling with an evolving paradigm in a town on the cusp of change. Some residents believed that science, government agencies, and Whirlpool would provide the protection that they expected. Yet others, albeit a small number, challenged the corporation and questioned the effectiveness of those institutions to effec-tively manage and respond to risk of toxic exposure. In many ways, impacted families' actions to resolve contamination were shaped and limited by the very forces they sought to challenge—science and unknowable risk.

The emergence of dissenting factions is a common occurrence within con-taminated communities, and in the case of Clyde, it is partly due to the ambigu-ity associated with the undetermined etiology of the disease cluster. Differing interpretations of environmental risk often underscore the conflicts that arise between groups.[39] Using the same sets of information about contaminated con-ditions, communities can splinter into opposing groups using different analyses to form opinions about risk. The contaminants are invisible, hence largely imper-ceptible, which further obscures their point of origin.[40] Regulating entities, such as state, local, or corporate management, exacerbate ambiguity either by withholding information entirely or presenting information that is contradic-tory. Consequently, affected residents must make corrective assessments of harm and decisions based on uncertain criteria.[41] As Auyero and Swistun observe, "diverse powerful actors' striking but contradictory claims about existing hazards shape the availability of information about the origins and effects of toxic contamination."[42] This affects how people make sense of and cope with toxic danger.

I argue that while human responses to environmental hazards are always mediated by interpretative processes, this mediation becomes more pronounced in the face of obfuscating information. Therefore, it is important to account for the cultural dimensions of rationality.

Values, norms, belief systems, and collective memories also play a role in how a community responds to residential toxic exposure. Mary Douglas was the first to argue that cultural, rather than individual, factors influence the ways that people make judgments.[43] From this perspective, the issue of resolving disagreements about risk is not related to correcting misguided perceptions and lack of knowledge, but rather is the result of differences in judgments on risk. A cultural approach is helpful in understanding communities like Clyde, Ohio, where most residents have taken little collective action even as multiple children and adults have been diagnosed with cancer.

When faced with emergencies that are not critically physical, most people respond with a diffusion of social responsibility, a "bystander effect" wherein we don't speak up because we assume someone else will take the lead.[44] Looking further upstream provides context to this insight. When our dominant culture promotes individuals as unattached, self-responsible market players, what follows is a rejection of any idea of responsibility—from the state toward individuals or from one individual toward others. Neoliberalism teaches through the socialization process that individual accountability and responsibility supersede the collective and "thoroughly revises what it means to be a human person."[45] Rather than looking at larger systemic or structural issues that might have caused widespread illness, the emphasis on individual accountability and responsibility infiltrated the community response to the cancer cluster and naturally segued into most individuals acting alone, disconnected from the community. Traditional and cultural values became eroded by market values.

While most political economists isolate the crisis of nature from that of finance and most ecologists similarly privilege the ecological dimension, environmental sociologists have tended to the dual crises of natural degradation and the disruption of social fabric. In addition to contradictions in capitalism internal to the economy (e.g., the contradiction between the notion that finance mobilizes and allocates resources efficiently and the reality of frequent finance-induced crises), noneconomic contradictions and forms of crisis also exist—what Nancy Fraser calls the social reproductive contradiction of capitalist society. Fraser defines these as the "human capacities available to create and maintain social bonds, which includes the work of socializing the young, building communities, of reproducing shared meanings, affective dispositions, and horizons of value that underpin social cooperation."[46] The debilitating processes of division in communities after disasters, as occurred in Clyde, is one such example.

The next chapter explores crises of social reproduction in Clyde—how neoliberalism is felt in the erosion of social relationships. I explore emotions in the narratives of Clyde residents during the period of acrimony in the community regarding the source of perceived environmental contamination, its appropriate remedy, and outcomes.

Emotion is embedded in risk discourses and strategies that reproduce inequalities and facilitate adaptation to instances of environmental risk. The threat of social ostracization by the pro-Whirlpool majority demonstrates how risk is used to reproduce and maintain concepts of selfhood and group membership. One becomes susceptible to othering by stepping outside that membership. I build on this literature by showing how emotion is implicated in social interactions and claims-making processes and in the social production of risk. I call into play Sara Ahmed's queries, 'What do emotions *do*? How do they work to secure the social hierarchy?' to advance an account of the work of emotion.[47] I examine othering as a set of processes that engender marginality and consider the implications of reading emotion in environmental disputes.

3 ▸ EMOTION, RISK, AND OTHERING

What moves us, what makes us feel, is also that which holds us in place, or gives us a dwelling place.

—SARA AHMED, *The Cultural Politics of Emotion*

WHEN CLYDE WAS classified as a cancer cluster, some residents suspected that Whirlpool was responsible for elevated rates of disease in the community. Perceptions of harm were amplified for some because of the profound impact on so many children, serving as the impetus for mobilization among affected residents seeking redress for the contamination. Those at the forefront of the lawsuit were more likely to investigate environmental concerns than were those not personally impacted. This group, as well as those sympathetic to the lawsuit, represented a minority of residents who dissented from the majority opinion regarding how to resolve the problem of cancer.

Family physicians and health department officials told families that the cancer cluster was likely linked to environmental toxins. After approximately seven years of frustration and failed attempts to achieve resolution through the Ohio Department of Health (ODH) and the Environmental Protection Agency (EPA), litigation seemed to be the only way to get answers and draw attention to the issue. The plaintiffs believed that attorneys and experts would advocate for them and take the lead in determining who was responsible for environmental contamination within the community. Plaintiffs emphasized that they did not have a particular agenda against Whirlpool, and that they did not want the company's Clyde plant to close. They simply wanted answers, and Whirlpool was not cooperating with their efforts toward finding them. The lawsuit was a last resort that they viewed as the only alternative in determining why so many people were getting sick. Plaintiffs knew that a lawsuit would allow them access to records and information in the discovery process that they would not otherwise be able to view.

Those in support of the lawsuit wanted Whirlpool to live up to its positive reputation within the community. If it were discovered that Whirlpool was responsible for cancer-causing pollution, they wanted the company to clean up the contaminants for which they were responsible and to prevent pollution from happening in the future, thereby protecting other residents from experiencing illness. They felt that accountability might even serve as a preventive measure in protecting other communities, as taking no action against the company might make other companies think that they could get away with similar offenses. Affected families also felt that they should be compensated for their losses. One father expressed a justifiable sense of advocacy for his sick children on both a financial and an emotional level in that they deserved to be supported not only for what they have been through but also for what could possibly happen to them in the future because of the consequences of their illness: "Our lives have been changed and their lives have been changed. We wanna find the answers and get to the bottom of it. However, if somebody or some corporation has done this, then I feel my kids deserve to have a better life in the future because their life may be one more year, may be five, it may be twenty. But there's a good chance they're gonna have problems down the road. So if [my kids were given] money from somebody, who caused something or did something, be it unintentionally maybe, I feel that they deserve a little break in life."

Most plaintiffs also believed that the legal system would help them find justice. In light of what was known about health consequences of PCB exposure, as well as the prevalence of disease within their community, there was optimism that some believed that the case would likely be ruled in their favor.

Yet there were powerful incentives for preserving the Whirlpool connection— not just preserving the source of employment for much of the town but protecting a long-cherished community identity as well. Conflict erupted between residents regarding the causes of the cancer. The group of affected families who were critical of Whirlpool's suspected complicity in the contamination was often met with condemnation by residents unwilling to criticize the company. Attempts at shaming plaintiffs were made through gossip, through repetition of rumor and threats, or by assigning blame upon them for endangering the sanctity of the town's identity, a narrative used to construct what is "normal" in the town. The congenial balance that had existed between town and corporation was threatened as residents became divided. The concept of normalcy shifted from the mere continuity of the town's comfortably beneficial patterns to a new "normal" defined by environmental threat, division, and health and economic concerns.

With connotations of "good citizenship" in their messaging, defenders of the company and the company itself claimed the moral high ground, which ultimately worked in the company's favor by undermining the plaintiffs. Sides were taken, but most residents chose to remain uninvolved. Despite approximately ninety calls to the EPA tip line, not one caller came forward to help the plaintiffs' case.

Collective mobilization is influenced by a community's prior industry presence, political involvement, experience with protest activity, and the collective civic capacity.[1] Emotion can stimulate or short-circuit individual and collective reaction to environmental crises within a community. Emotions such as pride, shame, and fear propel a politicized narrative and provide a script for residents— that they are only truly committed to the community if they align themselves with the company and against those others who threaten to take away the town's livelihood or identity.

PRIDE OF PLACE AND SHAME

Across a range of experiences, when one or more people achieve something positive or valued, the resulting feelings can be described as feelings of pride.[2] Scholars have made distinctions between being proud of one's personal achievements and feeling proud of the achievements of the group an individual belongs to or associates with.[3] Self-conscious emotions such as pride (or shame) require the evaluation of the self as superior or inferior and are determined with reference to socially valued outcomes.[4]

As it presents in affiliation with group identification, pride is a process that leads persons to see themselves as part of a group. Group-based pride depends on the degree of group identification and is shared with group members.[5] How one feels pride or shame when one feels group identification resides in the acquisition of "a social self or identity."[6] The group identity itself becomes personified and elicits pride or shame as a feature of that identity relative to the actions of that group.

Both bodies of literature indicate that pride is a status-related emotion with implications for identity and behavior. Henrietta Bolló, Beáta Bőthe, István Tóth-Király, and Gábor Orosz observe that the function of pride is to provide information about the social status and acceptance of individuals.[7] Self-pride serves an additional social function of motivating behaviors that are valued within an individual's social group.[8] Similarly, group pride is thought to motivate the pursuit of group-related goals and commitment to the group.[9]

Like pride, shame is a social emotion arising from viewing one's self from the standpoint of another. Sociologists view shame as an emotional response that we feel when we make a bad impression on others or fail to uphold our end of the social pact.[10] We feel shame because we have developed an identity as a "generalized other" and we feel accountable for societal prescriptions.[11] The experience or anticipation of shame usually induces a desire to neutralize that emotion or hide an aspect of the experience.[12] Symbolic interactionists understand this as a way we sustain the "integrity of the social fabric."[13] Social actors' efforts to avoid emotions like shame, guilt, and embarrassment reflect, create, and maintain social groups and hierarchies. Sociologist Thomas Scheff goes so far as to call shame the "premiere social emotion."[14] Whereas fear can be experienced irrespective of other people, shame always depends on judgments passed by other people. It involves reactions to rejection, feelings of inadequacy, and feelings of a threat to the social bond.[15]

A strong sense of pride permeates Clyde, a town where generations of families have lived. It was originally a farming community, and then a factory town, and its residents expressed nostalgia for what the town was like in earlier decades. Judy described there being a "real old-fashioned small-town atmosphere." There was an implication that "Americanism" was rooted in the fact that this country was built upon small towns like theirs. Some proudly referred to the town's nickname of "Little Chicago" because a secret underground speakeasy downtown served as a stopping point for notable Chicago gangsters during the Prohibition era.

From its inception in 1952 and even today, the Whirlpool Corporation has made a concerted effort to be viewed as a friendly neighbor with family and community values, a narrative that was also infused with ideals of the white suburban family. For over fifteen years, the communications section of the Industrial Relations Division presented a publication called the *Clyde-O-Scope*, which focused on employee and company activities in plant operations and in recreation. Some residents remember these publications as promoting family values and quality of life within the community.

Today, the influence of Whirlpool is evident everywhere in the town, reinforcing its importance to Clyde's identity. Community web pages describe the Whirlpool company with pride. The local library features a Whirlpool Room and a local community pub features a Whirlpool pork sandwich on its menu. In a 2017 *Toledo Blade* article titled "Huge Whirlpool Plant Runs Heart of Clyde," journalist Jon Chavez writes, "But the Clyde plant's significance is much more than wash cycles and spin cycles. Whirlpool has been a way of life in Clyde for five generations of families. The plant has spawned countless marriages, children, and friendships, not to mention a tax base that helps pay for roads and schools and draws business."

Clyde's mayor further noted that the "camaraderie and spirit in the plant derives from the relationships outside of it." These public texts are important in understanding how family and history are aligned and work to transform community relations with the Whirlpool Corporation into a familial tie. The family-culture narrative aligns family and history and works to transform transactional community relations with the Whirlpool Corporation into one of kinship.

Even prior to the opening of the pool at the park Whirlpool donated to the community, the imagined space would be one characteristic of the 1950s idealized family environment. The company limited access to the park to only company employees and their friends and families, which encouraged a sense of exclusivity that, in the words of one resident, "made outsiders want to be a part of it." A promotional video, created by Maytag and posted just a few months after the filing of the lawsuit against Whirlpool, provides an inside look at the factory facility with its waving American flag and is accompanied by a narrator who begins, "American pride is alive and well in Clyde, Ohio." The video then outlines Whirlpool's manufacturing successes before coming back full circle to the conflation of community with the company: "If you look at it another way, our community here in the plant is a big piece of the larger community outside our doors."[16] The company markets its heritage and family values in its other plant locations, too, and is one of many companies who use this trope as a marketing tool. Family-oriented themes are found in advertisements for a wide variety of companies—Hallmark, S. C. Johnson, Ford Motor Co. From greeting cards to cars, companies use their family-owned or family-operated status as a marketing asset, while others capitalize on simply the image of their products being sold in American stores or their products being used by families.

Whiteness is also implicated in the Whirlpool narrative and in the perpetuation of the community's identity as a perfect Middle-American town. Whiteness can be understood as an organizing principle. While many have noted that whiteness often operates as a taken-for-granted category, one of the most important contributions of the critical study of whiteness lies in "marking" whiteness as a particular identity, rather than as the presumed norm.[17] The symbolic meaning system of whiteness was repeated across generations in Clyde. Through the lens of labor history, David Roediger illustrates a linkage between the working class and whiteness and argues that the working-class identity is formed through othering.[18] This surfaced in quotes describing the town as a "safe" place to live in spite of the threat of toxic risk and contributed to assumptions of safety within the community.

Studies on coded language inadvertently support this idea. Scholars across a wide range of disciplines demonstrate that even when whites may not be aware of the racial meaning of their words, they use seemingly race-neutral terms that disguise explicit or implicit racial meaning.[19] References to the Clyde community were implicitly conflated with, and sometimes overtly expressed by residents as being related to, race and crime. The privilege of place, although unacknowledged, permeates these observations.

Suppositive identity led some to believe that they should have been safeguarded from disasters like contamination. Long-held ideologies about democracy, government, whiteness, and nationalism contributed to the frustrations some felt in assessing the dilemma. Marilyn, a sixty-four-year-old breast cancer survivor, exclaimed: "I'm supposed to be free," and "I'm an American—we're not supposed to live like this." She also voiced consternation in making the comparison to the 9/11 terrorist attacks, in that those events are commonly viewed as a collective American tragedy, while cancer clusters are not: "*We the people* are lost here somewhere. I don't know how you get it back. Do you have children die to get it back? After 9/11, everybody had a flag flyin' on their cars. Where are they at now?" Such expressions were accompanied by a sense of outrage that institutions of government had failed and their rights were being trampled on.

Even in conversations unrelated to the town's safety, the racial composition of the town was noted when identifying the town as having conservative values. "Generally, you feel safe here," noted one mother. "The school system has always been a really good school system, and I've never wanted to live in a big city so this is where I've stayed." Another resident observed, "People moved here 'cause it was nice, quiet—not that there aren't drugs in our town, but it was a little bit safer than some of the other towns."

Residents' impression of betrayal of the rights of "Americans" mingled with the perception that while other countries might face catastrophes like theirs, their own presumed insulation defined what was expected to occur. The conviction that cancer clusters were not something one would encounter in their town yet would be expected elsewhere indicate a presupposition that only "bad" communities would be expected to experience such harm. These mechanisms hampered activism as residents assumed protection from existing social structures.

Thomas Guglielmo emphasizes race as an ideology rooted in cultural and structural institutions.[20] While acknowledging that whites define themselves in relation to others, he makes an important point that they are already politically defined as white. With explicit attention to the centrality of the state, Guglielmo fills in a missing piece from Roediger's analysis—the role of white power and privilege. This insight is useful because it allows the meaning of whiteness to be conceptualized not only as formed with relation to others but as a form of capital. Other scholars, too, remind us that both whites and people of color live racially structured lives.[21] Whiteness infers a presumed status of unearned privilege that has afforded advantages in economic, educational, and social categories.

The insidious nature of toxic exposure provoked prolonged adversity in Clyde, a community that did not want to be marginalized as contaminated. It is predictable to have a strong response when people have an "attachment to current ways of working and do not want change to take place so close to home."[22] Betrayal of place and loss of trust in the existing social framework required renegotiation and self-examination. Karen and her parents, who lived near Whirlpool Park, expressed a feeling akin to grief as they reflected on what they described as "tarnished memories." As they recalled their children's and grandchildren's birthday parties at the park and their kids catching frogs in the creek, they wondered, "Were we safe or weren't we"?

Yet many persisted in their belief that existing social structures that favored them would hold. When sense of place is threatened, nostalgia is used to create identity continuity.[23] This was captured in comments made by residents like Carl who described a small-town atmosphere and whose best memories growing up included swimming at Whirlpool Park. Most residents in Clyde fell back into the safety net of a legacy system fueled by the desire to hold onto a treasured past. Thus, as seen in other cases of contaminated communities, the possibility of losing the valued town identity mitigated the probability of collective action.[24]

Erikson argues that in communities impacted by environmental disaster, people experience feelings of helplessness and depression that are in part a reaction to the thought that the community can no longer serve as a source of personal support—what he terms the "disaster syndrome."[25] But helplessness also contravenes the bedrock American principle of self-reliance and personal autonomy. Toxic contamination threatens the very idea of the American dream that promises a good life for all who are willing to work and abide by the rules. That a seemingly intractable problem like toxic contamination can take that away is difficult to accept, and the dissonance between fact and principle gives rise to a strong sense of unease that seeks emotional resolution.

Taken together, these examples of residents making sense of their community reinforce Thomas Gieryn's claim that place is a significant frame for interpreting their lives.[26] Importantly, though, they also illuminate rationales for understanding why othering is inherent in the meanings people attach to place and in their maneuvers to sustain it. There is a relational nature of the meanings people attach to "community," and the evaluation of the town as "valuable" enables it to become viewed as an object itself.

The communities of Clyde and Green Springs drew unwanted attention for being a "cancer cluster." A newspaper article with the heading "Cancer City, Ohio" was particularly stinging. Residents expressed feeling stigmatized by association with the tag "contaminated community" and shared stories of encounters with people from outside the community. "Oh, the cancer town," strangers would say.

One mother, whose daughter had died from cancer, reflected on the desire to protect the reputation of the town from the stigma of being labeled a cancer cluster. She observed, "You want to protect something that's your own. I have no idea why this example is coming to me—say that you were a wife who was beaten by her husband. Sometimes you'll defend him to the end and don't want to admit that he is what he is even though you know what he is . . . but you don't want other people to know that something's wrong."

While the mother's comment highlights the feeling of shame associated with the stigma of contamination, her analogy also evokes a spatial politics of fear.

Her analogy of stigmatization compared to a wife who is beaten by her husband conveys a gendered physical and bodily governance. It suggests a personification of the company as an aggressor to be protected despite of its transgressions, as occurs in many cases of domestic abuse. Reflecting a conflation of her individual experience with the community-level, her own self-surveillance is explained as a personal obligation to maintain the image of a "good" community.

FEAR

Fearfulness is mediated through a complex of physical, psychological, social, and cultural relations.[27] At an instinctual level, fear signals a threat to the body and can be experienced irrespective of other people. While fear originally evolved as an exclusively survival-based instinct related to self-sustenance, as society evolved, this was replaced by fear related to social status and relative well-being.[28] Thus, fear relates not only to the natural environment but to attributes of our social world. But fear also has a temporal dimension—the expectation of negative outcomes—and this makes it "more open to socially patterned processes of reinforcement and routinization."[29] In this way, fear can be understood as both primal instinct and socially constructed phenomenon, and examining the cultural matrix within which fear is realized can lead to insights on the patterns of social activity routinely associated with it.

While fear cannot exclusively be characterized as a primal instinct, it also cannot be understood as an exclusively socially constructed phenomenon. Joanna Bourke observes that there is a dimension of fear that is shaped by the interactivity between structure and agent.[30] Importantly, fear creates and perpetuates our institutions because it interacts with and acts on the social structure. The more widespread and prolonged the social anxiety, the more likely institutional change will take place.[31]

Mary Wrenn offers another novel way of thinking about it when she argues that if individual action and institutional evolution are truly interactive, then that should include the entire range of the human experience, including emotions.[32] At the individual level, people experience ontological insecurity, which is related to the need for social continuity and the ability to materially and socially reproduce one's standard of living. The fear of losing income or not having adequately funded and accessible health care, for example, means that some people are more ontologically secured than others. Those who are "more successful within the neoliberal project" are better equipped to suppress existential anxiety.[33] This framing allows us to understand fear as not only a private, individual experience but also as the shared experience of individuals living within the same sociocultural-historical context. There is a difference between anxieties felt at an individual level and those shared across a particular community.[34]

Several scholars have brought attention to the emergence of a "culture of fear" in late modern society.[35] Andrew Tudor builds upon these insights by offering a model that highlights the relations between the culture of fear and other aspects of modern society. Three of these parameters—environments, cultures, and social structures—refer to macroscopic features of the fear environment and play a constitutive and transindividual role in the construction of fear. What Tudor describes as "modes of institutional fearfulness" are interlocked with dimensions that are more microscopic in emphasis, relating to agency rather than structure.[36]

Fear manifests in diverse ways, but it is useful to consider how fear is structurally determined, how it provides a foundation for neoliberal ideology, and how it manifests in the practical effects on people subject to neoliberal power. For example, to the extent that the lack of regulation of environmental contaminants leads to environmental threats and illness, neoliberalism is implicated in the environmental mode of institutional fearfulness. In as far as neoliberal ideologies of individualism and its parameters for belonging are integrated into the attitudes, values, stereotypes, memories, ideas, and beliefs that are circulated within and through cultural institutions, neoliberalism is also implicated in the cultural mode of institutional fearfulness. Finally, to the degree that there is fear of company relocation or job loss due to economic downturns or mere social threats by managements, neoliberalism is also implicated in the social structural model of institutional fearfulness. Neoliberalism produces ontological insecurity through denying access to the means of reproduction and through existential breakdowns of financial failures. These fears in turn perpetuate neoliberalism as those who are able to turn to the market for protection or self-actualization.

How do we reconcile moral beliefs and commitments to helping our neighbors when our economic doctrines appear to put profit before people? With respect to inaction in contaminated communities and broader discussions about relational politics of contamination and neoliberalization, the politics of fear is an important and sometimes underestimated mechanism through which power expresses itself. Fear plays a central role in informing individuals of their place in the social hierarchy and, as such, reflects power relationships within a society.

Although fear cannot be directly mapped onto class, those less powerfully positioned experience more intense degrees of fear.[37] Limited access to financial resources limits their options in responding to threat. To exist on the perimeter of decision making where avenues of redress regarding one's own state of being are restricted, when those decisions directly affect one's own state of being, elevates a sense of helplessness that exacerbates fear. Therefore, while shame has been recognized as perhaps the most explicit "social" emotion, fear can also be understood as relational in the sense that it works to establish a relationship between subject and object.[38] It aligns subjects with collectives by attributing others as the source of their feelings. This is dependent on relations of power and creates distance between subject and object. As Sara Ahmed argues, it is more important to focus on what emotions "do" rather than on "what they are." It is through emotions, or how we respond to objects and others, that "surfaces or boundaries are made," as rejection from the collective norm implies that those othered lack worthiness to exist within the circle of the "valued" whole.[39] Emotion plays a central role in reproducing and maintaining concepts of selfhood and group membership.

While plaintiffs and residents alike lamented the stigma because of their shared pride of place, many viewed the plaintiffs and lawsuit against the company as the primary threat to the town's identity. Ultimately the plaintiffs' commitment to the community came into question as some expressed a sense of betrayal that the affected families, who had been previously supported by the community through multiple fundraisers, were going to "take the community down" with their lawsuit against the company.

This manifestation of fear in Clyde was related to an anticipated loss of employment. Standing up to the town's largest employer was a risk. As Marilyn explained, "People are afraid to say anything because they don't wanna lose their job. . . . It's a hard dilemma to put someone in—especially today." Because of this, some employees of Whirlpool who were ill themselves or had an ill child chose to remain anonymous. In fact, fewer than one-quarter of the families whose children had become ill or died were active in the lawsuit. They faced the dilemma of choosing between their family's health and their financial security and, for those who relied on health benefits from the company, these two considerations were interdependent. Beyond employee health benefits, losing work would mean not having money to pay for health care. As other researchers have found, residents were more likely to choose employment rather than face uncertainty.[40] And, as sociologists Shannon Bell and Stephanie Malin show in their research on the fossil-fuel sector, just as economic development and job creation goals can be used by companies to gain support, the same framing can divide communities and make it difficult to build support.[41]

Disengaged families also feared the consequences of standing up against the company. Stories circulated about employees being threatened for their participation in the public meeting, including an incident where an employee was approached and told, "You don't know who you're f-cking with." Information spread that an employee was reprimanded for speaking about the cancer cluster at a public meeting. A mother in one family with two leukemia-stricken children was told to minimize her family's media exposure. The fear surrounding employees who worked at the company was detectable when a man who worked there came home while I was interviewing his family and insisted on knowing who I was and what I was doing. "Just don't use *my* name," he said. He explained that he had been an exemplary employee and wanted to keep a low profile because his family needed him to have that job. His participation in the lawsuit also elicited concern from the man's coworkers, some of whom expressed disbelief that anyone would risk speaking out. He was told, "I can't believe you're doing that—they're gonna fire you. You better not turn your back on them." Stories such as these worked to the advantage of the company by stoking the fear of reprisal.

Rumors began to spread about repercussions from the company that perhaps also contributed to most employees' reluctance to speak about the issue. One such rumor created confusion regarding the legal right of stockholders to question the company. It was based on the idea that if employees were stockholders, they were legally bound to not speak negatively about the company. One man expressed concern that the company would retaliate by countersuing the plaintiffs for defamation. "That's why I say they'd better be darn sure. I would wanna be really, really sure what the evidence was before they went after somebody like *that*."

Suspicion arose that if the community turned on the company, management would relocate the company to another country. Their concern was not without merit. In 2010, although the company took approximately $19 million in stimulus money through the American Recovery and Reinvestment Act, Whirlpool relocated an Indiana refrigerator factory to Mexico in a move that cost the community approximately 1,100 jobs.[42] In 2012, the corporation closed a plant in Fort Smith, Arkansas, eliminating more than 1,000 jobs and again outsourcing its manufacturing to Mexico, a low-cost manufacturing region, where the implementation of the North American Free Trade Agreement has significantly weakened both labor and environmental laws.[43]

Taken together, these narratives of risk were expressive of the emotion of fear. Fear worked to align bodily and social space by keeping some from attending public meetings or speaking up about the culpability of the company. Fear in this case can be understood as a technique of governance.

DENIAL, APATHY, AND COLLECTIVE INACTION

Emotion plays a role in how people construct realities and then make sense of them. In studying the case of a Norwegian town whose very existence is jeopardized by climate change, Kari Marie Norgaard observes that awareness of a threat is not necessarily correlated with action, a pattern evident in other locales too.[44] One reason is that people are not capable of sustaining a state of anxiety over the long term, especially when they have no agency over the cause of or solution to a problem as complex, global, and seemingly intractable as climate change. Robert J. Lifton describes a "crisis of numbing" whereby living with the omnipresent possibility of disaster forces us to look the other way; otherwise we are gripped by an irresolvable crisis of powerlessness.[45] Norgaard calls this curious state "double reality": living with the knowledge of cataclysm alongside a "collectively constructed sense of everyday life."[46]

Norgaard examines how feelings of disconcertment, displacement, or anxiety and their opposite (safety, security, and belonging) work to uphold the social order and discourage dissent.[47] She notes that confronting environmental risk head-on is socially difficult because it requires questioning dominant norms that "everything is all right," that "we are good people who do no and deserve no harm," or that "our community and nation are safe." People may be aware of unfair distribution of health inequities, but when coping with guilt and helplessness, people use emotion management to suppress negative emotions, sometimes by avoiding thinking of them at all.[48]

The fracture created by toxic contamination in a community can generate confusion, perceived powerlessness, or indifference and can result in literally no response equal to the gravity of the problem.[49] There are numerous instances where eco-concern does not result in a common call to action. Hernandez examines how, despite recognition of contamination, risk is normalized and tolerance of risk grows when the threat to esteemed collective identity is challenged. In contaminated communities, identity is often rooted in a population's desire to perpetuate a history, an ongoing investment of space that has been positively nurtured over time. With the routine pursuit of daily life, they do the "important cultural work of making toxic life not only feasible but ordinary."[50] Similarly, Ahmed argues that emotions can attach us to the "very conditions of our subordination through our investment in social norms and their repetition."[51]

Alternately, expressions of shame and fear suggest another interpretation—a *denial* of the scope of the problem. One of the more vexing questions raised by the community's hostility toward the litigants was whether townspeople believed there was, in fact, a crisis at all. Although there was unquestionably a deposit of carcinogenic sludge festering beneath the park, coinciding with an anomalous spike in cancer diagnoses, residents' responses ranged from denial to dismissal to downplaying. Most did not accept that Whirlpool was at fault and offered other explanations for the cancer rates—lifestyle choices, God determining the course of one's life, or illness within the Whirlpool facility itself as an expected occupational hazard. Denial of fact enables suppression of the difficult emotions that acknowledgment of those facts might elicit. This "social organization of denial" occurs through a process of social interaction that dictates what should and should not be an object of our attention.[52] Not just fear but its *negation* or denial can be used as a mechanism of power, as occurred in Clyde. Denial is a cognitive rather than an emotional act that permits the suppression of negative feelings and the reinforcement of positive ones and emerges as another fault line in a splintered community. People process their relationship to risk through various emotional outlets. Denial is one way of neutralizing the fear that surfaces in the face of a significant threat. Another is sublimating it into an antagonism toward people who resist it. If those "resisters" are one's own neighbors, the emotional reaction can be particularly acute. Perhaps in a community like

Clyde, in the face of a breakdown of communal relations and the supremacy of the individual, these acts of resistance may have further eroded its own vision of itself as a "community."

In Clyde, as the breakdown of established interactions occurred, denial was particularly acute in that the community encountered challenges to its honorable image of itself. Attempts to consolidate the community were aggravated by acts of resistance considered to be divisive.

OTHERING IN CONTAMINATED COMMUNITIES

Othering is central to sociological analyses and cultural studies of how societies establish identity categories.[53] It is a concept that helps answer the question of how fear and risk are culturally constructed as products of social and economic systems that privilege those who "belong" over those on the margins. On a global scale, othering underlies systemic territorial disputes, violence, and military conflict.[54]

Acknowledging othering not just as an outcome but as integral to processes that produce and maintain difference opens the possibility of understanding inequality. Dimensions of othering encompass race, religion, sex, ethnicity, economic status, and disabilities. The process of othering initiates a standard by which members of one group contend their own worthiness while assigning negative traits to others.[55] Group-based othering gains social significance when challenges to the existing order manifest. Additionally, group-based identities central to conflict often expose preexisting grievances that emerge under stress.[56] As emotions are central to social order and group membership, one becomes susceptible to othering by stepping (or being forced) outside of the collective whole. In the context of environmental studies, William R. Freudenburg and Timothy R. Jones reference "corrosive communities" in which residents accuse and engage in harsh debate, leading to the disruption of the social fabric.[57]

What does it mean when one part of the body (whether corporeal or collective) is impacted while the remainder stays healthy? Often, in the aftermath of disaster, fault lines emerge between the affected and unaffected in a way that mimics preexisting inequalities and corrodes attitudes of unity. This kind of social "corrosion" is especially common after toxic events as opposed to natural disasters, where the aftereffects are immediate, obvious, and most likely to provoke an urgent and unified response.[58] Yet, even as one side tries to cleave from the other and escape the contamination, "traumatic experiences work their way so thoroughly into the grain of the affected community that they come to supply its prevailing mood and dominate its imagery and its sense of self."[59] Contaminated communities are often characterized by stress and anxiety as they come to grips with this eventuality, sometimes even splintering into opposing groups.[60] Divisions present when people are not capable of sustaining a state of anxiety over the long term, especially when they have no agency over the cause of or solution to a complex environmental problem. Freudenburg and Robert Gramling describe "diversionary reframing" wherein such groups engage in processes to discredit opposing groups.[61]

Othering, a demonstrative response to fear, is central to human subjectivity and offers a useful framework for understanding how emotions operate in people's lives. While group-based identities are complex and elude oversimplification, the consequences for out-group members subject to exclusionary tactics are costly. This can be seen in Clyde when the ascription of plaintiffs as fomenters of trouble and dissent amplified the perception of threat related to loss of community identity and employment. Processes of othering are both an effect of and productive of continuously negotiated relations of power.

Some community members also used coded language and diversionary reframing to discredit the plaintiffs by redirecting attention to the plaintiffs' personal beliefs and values rather than the contingent maladies present in the community.[62] Not only does the use of coded language allow the speaker to relate meaning without being specific, sometimes to hide their discomfort, but it is also used against a group or an idea that threatens traditional power structures. Coded language can similarly have as its subtext an indication of gender. "Emotion" has historically been conflated with weakness, as primitive, and as operating beneath the faculties of thought and reason. Gender scholars have shown how emotionality has been associated with femininity and works to subordinate women.[63] Among residents in Clyde, othering occurred when residents in Clyde insinuated that plaintiffs were emotionally misguided, implying that the reason some families filed the lawsuit against the company was because they were sad or angry and simply being reactive, and that the lawsuit would not bring their loved ones back:

> I don't know if it's right or wrong or if they're gonna accomplish anything or if they're just gonna you know hurt themselves in the long run because it's gonna take so much of their time and maybe away from their current family and their current lives, their involvement in their church, those kinds of things. That's the sad part, I feel for their families because I know like if the parents are really, really active in this and they're going to all these meetings and the other kids in the family seem to suffer a little bit because they're not you know going to their activities, they're not getting the current attention.

The presumption is that to be emotional is to have one's judgment affected. Claims such as these of emotionality *about* the plaintiffs, albeit couched in sympathy, endowed the plaintiffs with negative meaning and value by implying, for example, that their parenting skills were suspect, that their moral judgment was impaired. Comments such as these allowed complainants to criticize under camouflage of kindness and also, by contrast, cast their own position as morally worthy. Residents do the emotional work of othering with claims that themselves are emotional acts.

Assertions such as the explanation that the plaintiffs just "wanted somebody to blame" were rife with resentment. Similarly, the motives of specific individuals participating in the lawsuit were questioned and their worthiness regarding receiving financial support was scrutinized. Complainants implied that plaintiffs' incentives were predominantly pecuniary in nature.

The company's defenders also made strong appeals to "positive" emotions associated with home and community and even extended these to broader, deeper feelings about "American values." In this way, the company, in concert with residents who supported it, constructed a parallel emotional narrative that not only upheld a feeling of righteousness among the majority but ascribed negativity upon litigants, declaring an emotional division, a "moral disorder," between factions.[64] A spokesperson for Whirlpool also characterized the plaintiffs as the real threat when he said, "We will vigorously defend our company, our community, and our employees."

Claims of moral integrity were also embedded in comments about lifestyle risks, with the implication that illness among impacted residents was a consequence of choices they made. As genetics and lifestyle variables were largely attributed to the cause of cancer, many determined that the responsibility for controlling one's exposure to chemicals existed at the individual and family levels. Despite the uncontrollability of externally imposed environmental risk, the concept of self-monitoring was a described as a strategy for self-protection and one commensurate with "responsible living"—a caregiving responsibility.[65] One resident attributed the healthy lifestyle habits of her own family, for example, as the likely reason they have not been affected by disease. "I'm a firm believer in eating good food. None of us have any type of diseases like that. And I attribute it to food and keeping your mind healthy and busy and all that." A school nurse also expressed her firm belief that "eating healthy, exercising, and keeping your body well" are the key factors in staying healthy. She shared with me her own regimen for promoting wellness and recovery, and cited nutrition as the most promising avenue of cancer research.

A close reading of the work of emotions in Clyde illustrates that the narrative for critics of the lawsuit works through othering. Such others—the plaintiffs— threaten to take away what residents have. These are narratives wherein the plaintiffs are read as the *cause* of emotion in the very process of taking an orientation toward them. For example, when referring to the plaintiffs, one woman stated, "Once they made the decision to make us a cancer cluster and make that known to everyone, you can't take it back."

In Clyde, the process of exclusionary behavior leveled against the plaintiffs effectively relegated them to a status of other. Ahmed states, "If good emotions are cultivated . . . then they remain defined against uncultivated and unruly emotions. . . . Those who are 'other' to me or us, or those that threaten to make us other, remain the source of bad feeling."[66] In this way, emotional narratives reinforce social hierarchy and separate the degraded, uncivil, or "uncivic" feelings of outsiders. Othering can be thought of as a more severe *attribution* of shame and is deployed by members of a social group when shame is insufficient for getting people to adhere to the social order. It gains strength as the number of its practitioners reaches a critical mass: the more one's neighbors align with the dominant group, the harder it is to remain neutral or take the side of those being shamed.

The plaintiffs' lawyer, too, was perceived as being the *cause* of the town's stigmatization. After a public meeting, wherein the lawyer made a joke, albeit in poor taste, about the town's drinking water, a resident published a letter to the editor in the local newspaper. "Talk in the village has placed everyone on edge with continued attacks from a cowboy attorney now saying our village is built on a dumpsite and the water is poisoned." Such sentiments further reinforced the narrative that those outsiders (including the plaintiffs) who are "not us" threaten to take away what we (legitimate residents) have. The nature of civil action as a method of pursuing grievance also relocates the perception of autonomy from within the town to outside actors: attorneys, judges, and others working through a legal process that is distant, opaque, and slow-moving. This contributes to what Pamela Neumann calls "the use of experiential knowledge to contest the stereotypes and opinions of outsiders who are perceived as an existential threat to their community."[67] By labeling the plaintiffs as the *cause* of the town's stigmatization, the plaintiffs and their supporters' commitment to the community came into question. The company reinforced this framing of the problem by asserting its status as a caring "citizen" of the community. Many residents reiterated this by describing the company as a "good neighbor," suggesting the company would "feel hurt" that the community turned on them, thus ascribing constructing the company as a wounded subject worthy of sympathy.

Importantly, the governing power of fear is achieved through intensification of threats. "If the company goes, we would become a ghost town," a resident explained. Not only did plaintiffs threaten to stigmatize the town; they threatened to destroy it all together—"If Whirlpool left, our town would dry up and blow away." This had real consequences for plaintiffs who were confronted in public spaces—restaurants, hair salons, picnics—and experienced a social disciplining of which they were very much aware.

Dave, whose two children had leukemia, was challenged by an angry older resident who exclaimed, "I'm tired of this being all over the media and the circus. This isn't gonna happen to our town anymore!" These encounters made some families increasingly sensitive when going into town. Parents counseled their children not to voice their opinions for fear of social repercussions, including those from their teenage children's employers. When Karen's fifteen-year-old daughter got an interview at Pizza House, for example, Karen advised her to not voice her opinion to anyone she did not know.

Confronting disaster, especially disasters that are human produced, sometimes necessitates challenging norms. Those who demand redress are habitually maligned as contravening community values and are thus othered by those who see themselves as upholders of those values. These actions were advantageous for the preservation of a community's relationship with the corporation in question. In Clyde, what was hoped for by the plaintiffs in terms of remediation (or even symbolic justice) from a presumed corporate "good neighbor" was subordinated by their own neighbors who aligned with the company against them. The social processes involved in preserving the town's dynamic served ultimately to insulate the company, providing an example whereby the community itself works on behalf of the company, an operation of intimidation in which the residents themselves participate. If, in fact, Whirlpool were acting in good faith as the paternalistic good neighbor it contended it was, would it not work to address the problem it was suspected of causing? The question never needed an answer, as definitive responsibility for the contamination was never formally determined. Nevertheless, Whirlpool agreed to clean up the sludge in 2015. Because no specific source of the contamination was ever identified, the lawsuit was eventually withdrawn in 2015 and the plaintiffs received no monetary award from Whirlpool Corporation, even as cases of cancer among children and adults continued to present.[68] Despite the discovery at Whirlpool Park and anecdotal evidence of dumping at other locations in the community, residents have been unable to hold anyone accountable for contamination.

Regardless of where residents stand as to the cause of the cancer cluster within the community, those who were impacted experience continuing relative levels of distress and turmoil. No one has stepped in to find answers or correct the problem, nor has anyone been held accountable. The anxiety produced by human-made disasters is all the more distressing when other people, including one's neighbors and the individuals responsible, respond with indifference or denial. Residents have been left with few resources to solve the problem on their own, and consequently their versions of truth, community, and hope have been degraded. People who expected to live out their lives in a safe community now live with a heightened awareness of risk—both environmental and embodied risk.

The next chapter focuses further on ontological dimensions of neoliberalism as expressed and experienced by families impacted by disease. Building on classic work on communities in disaster, I detail the ongoing practical challenges of managing illness and the psychosocial effects of illness and contamination.[69] I consider how the climate of fear and marginalization impacts individuals' personal agency, identity, and psychosocial well-being. Having looked at how risk-related discourses marginalize the plaintiffs, in the next chapter I turn to how these discourses are negotiated or resisted by those who are the subject of them.

4 ▸ EMBODIED RISK

RISK IS CENTRAL to human subjectivity. Because the "facts" of toxic disaster are often unclear, the "perception" of the disaster becomes central to its effects. Despite efforts to interpret risk in absolute terms, these interpretations are always potentially unstable. "Risk-making" can occur along much the same lines as "race-making"—both can be characterized by processes that are socially constructed, fluid, and open to social and political influence. As illustrated by the division that occurred in Clyde, perception of environmental risk is consequential for action to occur.

It is useful to distinguish between environmental risks, lifestyle risks, and embodied risks. Environmental risks are those that exist outside the body. Lifestyle risks are those resulting from an individual's behavioral choices. In contrast, embodied risks are located in the body of the person said to be "at risk." Although they can be distinguished, these three types of risks overlap because the body can be affected by a person's way of life and also does not exist independent of the environment in which one lives. Ultimately, environmental risks and lifestyle risks cannot pose a threat without a vulnerable body.

These risks also have different consequences for the individual who is labeled "at risk." Environmental risks, although subject to varying perceptions, are generally thought of as externally imposed, rendering individuals as potential victims. Lifestyle risks may threaten the perceived moral integrity of an individual, as they are often viewed as being a consequence of something a person does. In contrast, for those who are living with embodied risk, the abnormality exists as a physical hazard within their body. Unlike environmental and lifestyle risks, an embodied risk holds a dual meaning—it is simultaneously a current illness and a signal of possible future disease or death.[1]

As such, embodied risks create unique problems. Whereas environmental risks can be interpreted as being externally imposed or something "done" to a person and lifestyle risks draw into question what a person "does or does not do," embodied risks impose their threat from within.[2] Experienced at a more personal level, embodied risk can become a part of who a person is, rather than what the person does or what is done to that person. People with disease can also come to experience their own body as potentially dangerous, prompting them to experience a division between body and self. Here, disease itself is the "other," conflated with destruction, invasion, and death. Being labeled "at risk" also involves medical surveillance and intrusion, as well as a great deal of ambiguity regarding the effectiveness of the steps taken to reduce the risk.

In Clyde, families impacted by disease faced challenges in accessing affordable health care, managing illness, keeping the family unit together during ongoing medical treatments, and maintaining a sense of normalcy. Fear was experienced as a response to trauma that in turn shaped the structure of their families. Anxiety about risk became routinized in their daily personal lives as they coped with the simultaneous presence of disease and the possibility of developing disease in the future.

SOCIAL, EMOTIONAL, AND PHYSICAL IMPACT OF CANCER ON CHILDREN

Because children require care, protection, and stability to thrive, the way they experience risk is fundamentally different from the way adults do. Their emotional and social development is more vulnerable to outside stressors and the denial of important opportunities that take a pause when a child is dealing with disease. While there are commonalities across the experiences of all youth, their experiences differ by age. Although it is a universal experience, the nature of fear is also not the same for everyone.

Chase Berger was four years old when he was diagnosed with cancer. After visiting his grandparents' house for a Halloween party, he returned home where his family noticed a bump under his right eye. It continued to grow, and after a series of doctor visits led him to an eye specialist, it was determined to be rhabdomyosarcoma, a soft tissue cancer. Chase was four years old when it was removed. His fifth birthday marked the first of many chemo and radiation treatments he would receive.

The initial days of medical intervention during which the child is often in the hospital are usually the most stressful for the child and the family. As a nineteen-year-old looking back on his experience, Chase noted his lack of awareness at the time of what could happen to him. What stood out to him in his early battle with cancer were the week-long chemo treatments and their side effects that led him to stay in the hospital for months. On top of dealing with their new schedule, Chase recalled the treatments making him so weak that he physically couldn't hold his body up and needed his mother's assistance. He shared, "My mom was always there pretty much controlling me because I couldn't control my own self because I was so weak and it was just really taking a toll on me."

Children encounter unique challenges during treatment for cancer. Because serious side effects do not occur as readily in children as they do in adults, children may be given greater doses of chemotherapy and radiation over shorter periods of time. Yet cancer and the side effects of treatments for the disease can often impact children more negatively than adults because of the harmful effects on developing organs. Side effects may occur immediately or appear years later. They have the potential to affect a child's growth or even cause a second cancer to form. Children may also respond differently to drugs that control symptoms in adults. Leukemia, lymphoma, or a cancer or treatment that affects the central nervous system (the most common cancers affecting the children in this study) involve consecutive, often invasive and painful medical procedures. Lumbar punctures (LPs) and bone marrow aspirations (BMAs) which are administered to children with leukemia, for example, have been identified as a major stressor for children because of the pain associated with those treatments.[3]

Along with apprehension about receiving repeated, often painful medical care, being away from their familiar home environment is a common fear for young patients. Medical surveillance and technologies change the spaces kids inhabit and how they conduct their day-to-day activities, build relationships with others, and come to an understanding of who they are and the world they live in. While being home from the hospital may make things feel more normal, the constant subjection to technologies used to track and monitor their disease often extends into the home as families assume treatment duties. After his hospital stay, Chase's mother was shown how to administer his shots at home.

The Hisey family's experience also illustrates some of the unseen challenges associated with the familial management of cancer. Tanner would spend weeks lying on the family couch because he did not feel well after the completion of his treatments. Because a port was implanted in Tanner's chest to provide an easier way to receive medications and have blood samples taken, steps had to be taken at home to prevent infection and to care for the port.

As the home environment is adapted for patient care, the social environment for children with cancer also changes. Contrary to literature that shows no differences in measures of social isolation between children with cancer compared with other healthy children, parents often perceived changes in their children's social relationships. Alexa's father, Warren Brown, for example, remembered observing the moment his daughter realized that she was different from other children, and that she would be different from then on:

Alexa used to go over to the neighbor's house and jump on their trampoline with the other girls. I remember. This was after she got out of the hospital, after her surgery, after learning to walk and talk again, and keep in mind Alexa's gait was never the same ever again. She could never have walked normally again I don't think. Maybe over time, had she had more time, she would have strengthened those muscles and become a little more agile, but she stood at the dining room window and looked across the street at the girls jumping on the trampoline. And that's when it hit me that [pause] she knew she would never be the same again, she knew there were something different that would always be different that . . . just from her body language, from the look from her face, I was struck with the fact that it's never gonna be the same for her.

Typically, at the onset of learning about one's chronic illness, young children may not fully comprehend chronicity. What Alexa's father was describing was a sort of reconciliation of Alexa's self to illness as she seemed to acknowledge her new limitations alongside a sense of feeling trapped within an ill-functioning body.

Although the experiences of youths with cancer are undertheorized in the literature, interviews with the families in Clyde suggest that there are similarities and important differences between children and adults in how chronic illness affects self-image. One similarity is that, like adults, older children might initially be able to maintain the same image of self, not allowing disease to become an essential part of who they are. Only through time and interaction with others do the meanings of disability and impairment become real.

Young adults and adolescents are especially at risk of distress, depression, and anxiety. When their lives become more organized around the demands of illness, it is common for them to turn inward, to become more socially isolated, and to begin questioning their emerging identity. For teens during this transitional life stage of adolescence, the effects of disease can contribute to a loss of independence, which is particularly important to them. Young adults have the desire to pursue independence in order to construct their identities, yet this independence may no longer be available to them. Like adults, many youth with cancer view themselves as physical as much as mental beings and therefore any change in body image is significant. Embodied risk is thus inextricably tied to changes in one's sense of self. The diagnosis of disease redefines them as being "at risk" as chronic illness undermines their ability to take for granted a well-functioning body and disrupts a sense of wholeness between body and self.

Some people with chronic illness become disabled, but some do not. Disabilities may result from chronic illness, but they also may be traced to trauma, accidents, injuries, and genetic disorders.[4] Children who experience damage to motor skills or even disfigurement from cancer treatments that require corrective surgeries may have a permanently altered physical appearance and face monumental challenges both physically and socially. Survivors of pediatric cancers that result in physical impairment have been found to be less likely to have completed high school, ever worked a job, or ever been married.

The adjustment of people with a chronic illness or disability can be very much influenced by the manner in which they are treated by others. Poor body image may lead to low self-esteem and can affect the ability to form healthy peer and intimate relations. In studies on peer relationships and adjustment, children with cancer have lower satisfaction with athletic competence than their peers. Dave described the physical changes his son was experiencing due to treatments, citing how his classmates were sprouting above him as he "missed out on all the social things through junior high." Tanner's sister and mom also reflected on his difficulty with this issue:

SIERRA: I think one of the biggest problems for Tanner was his friends, because he was always behind. I was almost taller than Tanner, and I was what, 4, no 5 foot maybe? And I was almost taller than Tanner when he was going into high school. He was super small, and all the girls friendzoned him.

DONNA: He's a sweetheart.

SIERRA: He's the nicest kid you would probably ever meet to a girl and I mean they just always kept him that way. He was always self-conscious. The girls thought he was too short, all this other stuff. He goes, "All my friends are older than me and they're playing all these sports I can't play 'cause I was too" . . . and he's still hesitant to tell people about it. Like I almost slipped up and told somebody when he didn't want it and he's like "oh!"

Stigma is social. When others view an illness or disability in a demeaning manner, they impose a stigma or discrediting label on the individual. As Tanner's story illustrates, adolescents might experience internalized shame and feelings of being set apart from others who are well. Needing to maintain secrecy about their illness, they might experience feelings and loneliness and detachment. They might not want to be socially identified and self-defined exclusively by disease, or at least may not want to bring attention to that part of their identity among peers.

Yet adolescents have different experiences with adaptation to disease. While Tanner experienced changes in his social relationships, Chase expressed "never having issues with making friends or his friendships changing" because of his history of cancer. He felt this way despite having had his eye sewn halfway shut in first grade because it wouldn't completely close at night due to the radiation he received. The doctors hoped that doing this would train it to close on its own all the way, although it never was completely remedied and remains sewn. Even though now Chase is a young adult, he has adapted to living with his impairment by adapting to the experience of it. As a high school football player, he acknowledged that not being able to see out of his right eye as he ran on the left side of the field or tried to catch a football affected him. But he explained, "The way I look at it is if I'm going to play a sport and I'm going to do it, I'm going to do it just as good as everybody else. I'm just the same normal kid. Yes, I might have my eye sewn shut and I can't see out of it, but that's not an excuse. That's just kind of the way I look at it. I mean, it is being hard on myself but, at the same time I'm just, that's kind of how I've adapted to it."

Children with cancer may also experience changing relationships at school simply due to the challenges of absenteeism. Dave Hisey reflected on how his children missed out on physical, social, and cognitive development, as well as things that would have been important to them in the course of a normal childhood, from missing school. Tanner lamented missing out on playing sports and other social activities due to his implanted port. These were also missed opportunities for social skills development.

Falling behind in academics was particularly stressful for Dave's son. Oftentimes, when his son was home from the hospital, he would be so ill from the side effects of his treatments that it further delayed his ability to catch up with schoolwork. This would result in him having a large amount of homework when he finally started feeling better, creating another layer of consequence to an already difficult experience.

Therapies that affect the central nervous system increase the risk for cognitive effects, which can lead to a wide range of short-term and long-term learning problems that include problems with memory, difficulty focusing, and difficulties with hand-eye coordination.

Clyde schools were supportive and created necessary accommodations for sick children to assist with their unique needs. The school nurse explained how radiation treatments to the head could cause traumatic brain injury, and how most of the kids diagnosed with cancer were on Individualized Education Plans (IEPs). Additionally, when children were absent for a long period, they were put on an IEP so that they could be given accommodations to meet the child's educational needs, such as allowing for additional time to complete class work. In Chase's experience, because he missed more than seventy-five days of first grade, he was held back.

Returning to school after treatment can provide a sense of normalcy, albeit in a slightly altered form, for children. The perception of the school nurse Nancy was that parents of sick children wanted them to be in school to normalize their children's lives—to "be at school and do what kids do at school." Children with cancer often demonstrate an eagerness to go back to school after treatment, but upon returning to school can face difficulties in psychosocial adjustment in the areas of scholastic capability, emotional stability, and social competence.

The school nurse observed that affected children were initially more needy and insecure when they returned to school, and that they "had a lot of fear wondering if they were really cured." At age eleven, Tanner had a greater awareness of the possible outcomes of his disease compared with younger children. His family would learn that Tanner said goodbye to his classmates in anticipation that he might not live. Sometimes the school nurse identified psychosomatic illnesses among the impacted children and would redirect them to the guidance counselors. In terms of identity, this seems to suggest that those with illness come to think of themselves as ill—an identity that lasts for some time post-treatment.

Another symptom of anxiety appears in the form of sleep disorders in affected children. Dave described his son's experience: "He, he always wants to be around someone, sleep with somebody because he doesn't want to be alone by himself, and that's gotten so much worse over this. And, you know, he's gonna be fifteen and I feel bad for him about that, you know? But on the other hand then you want him to be close to you so you end up caving because you don't know what next week's gonna bring."

While cancer survivors experience difficulties, some studies have shown that this anxiety typically decreases over time, and that most children treated for cancer, as well as children who are long-term survivors of cancer, have few serious psychological problems, even if physical problems persist. In general, children may experience high self-worth, good behavioral conduct, and improved mental health and social behavior upon cancer treatment completion. Quality of life for children with cancer is also strongly correlated with parents' self-efficacy, as well as parental responses to stress and coping.[5]

PARENTAL LOSS OF CONTROL, HELPLESSNESS, AND FEELINGS OF GUILT

Children with cancer are at elevated risk for adjustment problems. But when a child is diagnosed with cancer, adjustments are also made by their parents. The emotional consequences of cancer diagnoses introduce families to new, unwelcome feelings of fear, sadness, uncertainty, and a sense of responsibility. Parents experience fear and worry with relation to their child's potential fatality and to whether their treatment will lead to a full recovery. Parents' perception of their ability to positively influence the child and his or her environment can affect the child's adjustment. Parent vulnerability can also be tied to other factors such as education levels, resiliency, or having a child with poorer diagnosis, and may contribute to the ways parents cope with this stressful event.

I first interviewed Dave Hisey at his home in June 2013. He reflected on moving from Indiana to Clyde where he met his wife, Donna, and married her shortly thereafter. Like many others, he had a positive first impression of Clyde as a family-friendly place where he would want to raise kids. He described himself as a fun and loving parent with a life that revolved around his family, traits that were on display during our interview as he interacted playfully with his daughter Sierra, who interrupted to request permission to go to Twistee Treat, the local ice cream shop, to meet a friend.

Dave spoke candidly with me as he shared stories that illustrate the anxiety, emotional, and financial difficulties that accompany the tremendous burden that disease can place on a family. In February 2006, the Hiseys' daughter Tyler was diagnosed with AML leukemia and underwent seven months of chemotherapy at Saint Vincent's Hospital in Toledo. Dave recalled how the shock of diagnoses of his children disrupted the expectations they had about their lives. "We were just thinking that life was just starting, you know? Not thinking about kids' lives ending," he explained. Similar expressions of shock were echoed as families independently and collectively recalled the smallest of details surrounding the traumatic discovery of their loved one's cancer. Many in Clyde described having to quickly adjust to a "new normal" as interactions with the medical community became a predominant feature in their lives.

Dave and Donna wanted to take an active part in the treatment-related care of their daughter. Studies show that most parents, although less qualified to assess treatment options at the time of diagnosis, are better situated even than professionals to assess their child's pain level.[6] Taking a passive role in the decision-making process for their child's treatment can restrict parents' sense of control and autonomy.[7] At the same time, Dave and Donna also wanted to keep their other two children's lives as normal as possible. To counter the disrupting situations their kids were in, Dave and his wife tried to maintain a positive home atmosphere and retain a sense of normalcy.

> Everything else has been taken away from them so we wanted to do everything we could to keep home the same because they're in the hospital and when they come home we wanted them to come home to the familiar because everything else was different. They pretty much grew apart from their friends because you don't have all that contact with them every day, you know, and even when you do get back to school, people treat them differently or they're different, you know, they don't have hair, they're sick a lot and miss a lot of school. So, home was important to us.

In an effort to reassert parental control, they reshaped their role by focusing on their children's physical and emotional needs. Yet the bureaucratic aspects of managing illness, which included having to travel outside of town for treatments, led to a temporary displacement of their family and rearrangement of their parent roles. It was decided that Donna would stay with Tyler at the hospital to "be there" for her, while Dave would stay with their other two children at their home in Clyde in an attempt to continue "regular" lives that were centered on homework and sports.

But splitting duties and separating to care for their sick daughter at the hospital and the two other healthy children at home, with its disruption to family cohesion, placed an undue hardship upon their family. On top of adjusting to the cancer diagnosis, parents experienced role overload, which refers to an imbalance between the role demands placed on the individual and the resources at the person's disposal to meet those demands.[8]

Donna Hisey spent nearly all seven months that Tyler was in the hospital at her side. In addition to missing informal day-to-day parenting and family time at home such as monitoring, direct skill and knowledge instruction, providing guidance, and giving encouragement, parents also give up social roles and may become isolated from interpersonal relationships while caring for their sick children. Just as their children's friendships change, many adults experience disruption among their own friendships. Those involved in the lawsuit felt this. One parent reflected, "Sometimes some of your friends will stay away from you, you know, through it. But most of your friends you know still associate and stuff like that. I do feel some pushback."

Mothers of children with cancer may experience alienation and loneliness as they surrender some of their roles at home and in society to care for their child. Studies find that mothers caring for their children experience anxiety, depression and, compared with other family members, experience a higher level of post-traumatic stress symptoms.[9]

Though not all families were split between living at the hospital and home, many had to travel repeatedly for care, which was itself a stressful event. Chase Berger and his mother, only twenty-two at the time and who played an almost exclusive role in his care, woke up at three o'clock in the morning to make the one-hour-and-thirty-minute drive to the Cleveland Clinic. Again, unavailability of health services within or near the community was a burden that required uncomfortable adaptations to time and place.

Unexpected emergencies during a child's treatment also led to anxiety among parents. After leaving the hospital after three months, Chase recalled being at a family gathering when he began to feel hot and cold. Although they did not know this at the time, Chase's body was reacting to an infection. His mother drove him to the nearest hospital where he began to hallucinate. Because the doctors at the local hospital were unable to help him, he was life-flighted to the Cleveland Clinic, where physicians informed his mother that it might be the last time she would see Chase. Chase would recover but required several more months of hospital care to restore his health.

From this point on, Chase's mother started staying at the Ronald McDonald House, which helped alleviate the financial burden of fuel and lodging expenses. At a time when a family's focus needs to be on caring for their child and their own well-being, the financial toll of cancer treatment is nonetheless immense. Many families are forced to take time off work to care for the sick child. Even after treatment, a child's immune system may be so compromised that the child cannot return to daycare or school, which also requires the parent to find an alternative arrangement for childcare or stay home themselves. Such socioeconomic circumstances may undermine parental self-efficacy and affect parenting practices.

Uncertainty about treatment and outcomes, coupled with external barriers to care, elevated the level of strain experienced by parents. It also affected their self-efficacy, an affective component of the self-concept that is defined as the perception of oneself as a causal agent in one's environment.[10] While self-efficacy can be understood at the micro level as it is created and reproduced through individual and group-level processes, it can also be understood as the outcome of larger structural forces such as availability of and access to quality health care, paid and unpaid work, and the health of the neighborhood where one lives. These social structures affected not only parents' sense of control but also their mental health. Self-efficacy itself affects the physiological stress response, as well as the adoption of behaviors that are related to health outcomes, illustrating that the self-concept not only is socially produced but, in turn, can be understood as a social force. Low self-efficacy, or loss of control, can also impact behavior in the various institutions to which we belong, including the family.

Family cohesion can be strengthened by family members' experience with childhood cancer, but more frequently the preexisting family order is challenged. Many parents may view their spouse as the most important source of social support, although perceptions of support from spouses and assessments of marital quality decrease when the number of the child's hospitalizations increases.[11] Studies show that this is, in part, due to the wife's perceptions of support from her spouse being related to the husband's involvement in the care of the child, while the husband's perception of support from his spouse is related to the wife's availability in the home as opposed to the hospital.[12] In reflecting on the various dynamics of marital stress in the face of a child's diagnosis, Dave explained,

It does gnaw away at you with just all the different little things that you wouldn't really think about. . . . I mean it just affects everybody differently. Doctors said lots of people get divorced through it and we would've thought "Ah that'll never happen" and, I mean, marriage is hard enough without throwin' all that stuff in. You'd think it makes you grow closer, but it's just there's so many decisions and how to handle things. When Donna and Tyler were up at the hospital, ya know, we weren't there enough, we didn't call enough. We were gonna keep things normal at home, but it's one thing to say that, but then when they're stuck up there at the hospital feeling isolated and by themselves and we talk to them on the phone and then we wanna get off quick ya know (pause) and it's hurtful to them and it's . . . yeah, it's amazing. I was talking to the Browns the other day and I think people don't understand the whole thing they just look at the sickness.

Warren Brown acknowledged that this type of experience can fracture families because it is very easy to start "playing the blame game." In reflecting on the course of his child's cancer, he, as other parents, wondered if he could have controlled any circumstances which would have made a difference. He explained: "What else could we have done? Where else could we have taken Alexa for treatment? What did we not do that we could have done? And all those blame games could easily have crept in, and, to some degree we did start down that road at one point in time—the whole family. . . . There were times when there were very heated discussions about why didn't we do this and why didn't we do that. But in total, the loss of Alexa has drawn our family unit much closer together than we ever would have been."

Some parents expressed personal feelings of guilt and even implicit expressions of self-blame related to the onset of their child's diagnosis. It was during the summer of 2008, when Dave and his wife were coaching their son Tanner's baseball team, that Tanner began complaining about his arm hurting. He had some blue marks on it and was frequently tired. They did not think much of it, but they did have a couple of blood tests done which came back negative. After his third practice of Peewee football in the late summer, Tanner came home and complained, "Dad, I'm always so . . . I'm really hurt." Dave recounted how he affirmed that what his son was experiencing was normal. "It's just growing pains, Buddy. You're just working hard with practice. All the guys are with you on that. Push yourself, work hard." Still, they took Tanner to the hospital, where a lump on his neck was discovered, removed, and determined to be cancerous. The unimaginable had happened again. Two years after his sister's diagnosis of AML leukemia, Tanner was diagnosed with T-cell lymphoblastic leukemia at the age of ten. He underwent four years of chemotherapy. Dave lamented his initial lack of response to his son's complaints about not feeling well.

Parents strived to render their children's diagnoses intelligible. Their interpretation of their child's cancer was drawn from their broader understanding of cancer, as well as widespread medical and popular discourses that emphasize risk avoidance and personal accountability. Some mothers viewed their own bodies as sites that bear and transfer risk, and their actions and choices become central to mediating risk. In making sense of her daughter Alexa's diagnosis, Wendy conceptualized her own susceptible body as the possible source of Alexa's vulnerability, identifying hazard within her own body and then putting forward her environment as a possible cause of that hazard. She wondered if her daughter's cancer was something she had "passed on to her" from her own years of swimming at Whirlpool Park, expressing suspicion that chemical risks resided within her own maternal body or that there was something wrong with her body. Alexa's mother, Wendy, recalled not having belonged to Whirlpool but having friends who took her there and spending a lot of time there. She continued, "So then you wonder, 'Okay, is this something that could have gotten into my molecular cell structure?' Because Alexa never, *she* never went swimming there. The other kids—they went there, but Alexa never went swimming there. So then you wonder, 'Is it something that *I* passed on to her?'"

Parents also experience guilt that their parenting decisions may have affected the progression of the disease. Echoing public health discourses that emphasize individual choices, Wendy continued:

> We didn't get into the nutritional aspect with her until the year she died—with a nutritional specialist that treated brain tumor patients . . . different antioxidants and supplements and things. And so by the time she was . . . well, a month maybe before she died . . . I mean, she had a list this long of things she was trying to take . . . she was trying to . . . that would help her get better. But we didn't start those until January. I mean there again with another thing . . . you find out things that you shouldn't be and should be and if we had started that sooner . . . who knows if it would have made a difference.

Loss of control extended beyond the inability to control disease or its consequences. While levels of concern about the safety of their environment varied among participants, impacted residents were more likely to question the safety of everything around them. Some parents questioned their children's prior activities, searching their memories for possible links to exposure. There was heightened anxiety related to the source of contamination and the resulting inability of parents to protect their children in the face of the unknown. Furthermore, exposure to toxins is "psychologically burdened with legitimate expectations of the worst outcomes." This process of catastrophization, or believing that catastrophe is imminent, can itself be understood as an anxiety disorder.[13]

Guilt was compounded by a sense of helplessness in their limited abilities to know what had initiated the cancer, in their inability to affect the child's treatment, as well as in the length of the treatment period. This sense of helplessness challenged one of the primary roles of parenthood—that of being able to protect their children.

THE IMPACT ON SIBLINGS

Siblings of children with cancer often experience the same conflicting feelings that parents do as they observe and experience changes within their family. Siblings also engage with tasks such as visiting the hospital for treatments and become familiar with medical concepts and procedures. They may even exhibit stress responses to the illness experience themselves, including difficulty sleeping and complaints of somatic symptoms.[14]

For his siblings, Bubba's diagnosis unsettled a previous understanding of him and themselves as somehow immune to external threat. Jacob James "Bubba"

Andrews died on March 18, 2012 from glioblastoma multiforme at age twenty-two. He was a popular "superstar" athlete in Clyde and was recognized for his athletic ability outside Clyde as well. Bubba's siblings described him as a protective caregiver who sometimes helped their single mother and stepped into a somewhat paternal role within their family in the absence of their father. "He was the dad," his siblings explained. As I sat with his family by the pool of his sister's apartment complex, they fondly recalled how people throughout the state would refer to them with reference to Bubba. "I've always been 'Bubba's mom,' and these are 'Little Bubbas,'" his mom laughed. His youngest brother chimed in: "'Little Bubba #7' was on the back of my hat the first year I played for the Merchants." In reflecting on the diagnosis of their son and brother, Bubba's family remembered the drama surrounding the discovery that Bubba was sick, recalling the meeting with his doctor, and the very moments they were told that Bubba had had a seizure and was in the hospital. "He was just so healthy, and just a normal kid. Never got the flu, never got a cold," his sister recalled. One of Bubba's brothers added, "He was more than a normal kid. He was Superman."

On the one hand, Bubba's siblings described Bubba as initially being in denial about his diagnosis. His sister recalled that Bubba had a "very good ability to zone out at doctor's appointments and escape from reality by not paying attention to exactly what they were saying." However, his family suspected that he privately struggled but did not want his family to feel sorry for him. It was easy to deny Bubba's condition for a while because he "looked normal." His mom recalled rushing home from chemo treatments so that Bubba could go golfing or play in a softball game, and he would be concerned about not being home quickly enough. His sister, who had recently graduated from college, was scheduled to start working at a new job in a new city the week after he was diagnosed. "At the beginning, it wasn't quite real," his sister explained. As his tumor began to spread, however, his family confronted the reality that he would die, and the family supported Bubba as he grew more ill.

Like parents, healthy siblings of a child with cancer must cope with new logistical and social changes in their family. When Bubba began chemo treatments in Columbus, he lived with his sister, who took him to his treatments and tried to be there for him in any way that he needed. He maintained the protective role he played in his family until his death, at times even helping his mother cope with her sadness. She reflected on how he gave strength back to her—how he helped her understand that she needed to appreciate the time that they had together, rather than anticipating the end.

Sierra Hisey, whose two siblings had leukemia, also filled more roles at home, including tending to Tanner when he was sick on the couch, fetching things that he needed, and putting washcloths on his face. These tasks were not imposed upon her, but rather something that she undertook herself to provide support for her brother. Fulfilling additional household-related tasks and caring for sick siblings decrease time and availability for children participating in social activities outside the home. As for parents, these new tasks may also lead to role overload and chronic stress for siblings, as well as a conflict between their desire to resume their routine peer-group lifestyle on the one hand, and the role they undertake or are expected to undertake to compensate the sick sibling for his or her inability to participate in the peer group's social events and routine, on the other hand.[15] Sierra reflected on this time: "I still don't feel like I had a childhood. Like, I never went out. I never hung out with my friends other than family friends that were friends with my mom and dad. That's it. I never went to anybody's house; I never spent the night. I stayed with [my family]."

Healthy siblings may understandably spend less time with parents who are otherwise engaged with the care of the sick child and their special needs. While healthy siblings worry about their sick brother or sister, they might simultaneously perceive the distribution of attention as being unequal, leading to feelings of resentment and exclusion.

At the same time, just as Bubba's mother acknowledged the role of her children, including Bubba himself, as being socially supportive, Dave Hisey noted that his children also seemed to have increased empathy for him and his wife, and they would often try to lift their parents' spirits if they detected sadness in them. While acknowledging the important role of family and friends in providing support, Dave described the caregiving roles that his children assumed for their parents: "Believe or not, the kids were a big support—even the sick ones. Sierra would cheer you up when she sees you down because of Tanner. You know, Tanner—even though he was sick, seeing Mom and Dad upset, he would try to make you laugh. Somehow you can say the kids are a big part of the support, I think."

Healthy siblings expressed that their own friends were initially very supportive. However, as their sick sibling's disease progressed, those friends began to fall away, possibly because they did not know how to be supportive. Bubba's siblings reflected on this within a broader conversation about how the process of Bubba slipping away was painful and long for the family. Still, Bubba's siblings described how the relationships they had with each other since Bubba was diagnosed had solidified. "We have never been closer in our lives," his brother explained to me.

Dave also described the respect that his children developed for each other, and the increased compassion and empathy that his daughter Sierra had developed for others more generally. From his perspective, the experience of having two sick siblings had prompted her to mature at an early age.

The impact of Bubba's death affected his siblings and how they viewed themselves in different ways. While each had different ways of staying connected to Bubba after his death, one brother described how he honored Bubba by emulating his diligence, his work ethic, and the same approach to life that Bubba had. "From that point on we knew for all of us that we had to be better than we were to make up for what he was gonna be missing," he explained. All of his siblings described valuing life more and having an overall increased appreciation for living. Yet Bubba's sister struggled with feelings of anger over her brother's death: "I'm sad obviously because I don't have my brother anymore, but I'm more mad at the fact that this had to happen to him. I have had a lot of struggles with it, and you know, I am not the same person I was before this happened . . . not necessarily in a good way because it just . . . it really messes with your head and your perspective on life."

His youngest brother expressed feelings of survivor's guilt and compared himself to the type of person Bubba was, as if that were a factor in why some people get cancer: "I always thought, why not me? Why him? He was always the best at everything. The best at sports, he was better in school. . . . I just felt like the world would have been better off with him instead of me."

These emotional burdens were connected to a fear present among healthy siblings that they would also become ill. Bubba's sister reiterated, "It really really messes with your head." Dave and Donna's daughter Sierra often wondered if she, too, would be impacted by leukemia like both of her siblings were.

THE TRICKLE-DOWN BURDEN OF HEALTH CARE

Since its early years, America's health-care system has been based on a private market approach. The laws of supply and demand that functioned in other areas of the economy were also considered appropriate for the health-care system. This competitive foundation has stimulated the development of superior medical schools, innovative medical technologies, and the highest quality of health care possible. Yet despite spending more than all other wealthy democracies on health care, millions of Americans struggle with expensive bills because the government does not restrain the costs of insurance premiums, co-payments, deductibles, prescription drugs, and long-term care. The management of chronic illness and the high cost of medical treatments it requires can be financially devastating for families, leading households to make financial choices between health care and basic living expenses. These barriers also lead people to make unhealthy care decisions, limit their consumer choice, and increase costs to the health system.

In the living room of their small trailer, Donald and his wife, Shelby, spoke with me about the financial struggle of being on multiple medications, being unemployed, and being ineligible for disability benefits. Donald, a fifty-two-year-old former factory worker who spent much of his childhood in Clyde and Green-Springs, was in remission from chronic myelogenous leukemia (CML) and also had a kidney removed due to an additional unrelated tumor. For the first three years of being sick, Donald held a salaried position in quality control, and with the allotted vacation time, he was able to conceal his health status from his employer by taking time off when he was sick. When the economy declined and he lost his salaried position, he could only find jobs with hourly wages that did not provide sick days or insurance. Like others with chronic illness and disability who worry about job security due to workplace discrimination, Donald was concerned that if potential employers knew about his condition, they would not hire him out of concern about insurance increases.

Although Donald was in remission, he had to take the medication Gleevec every day. Every time his bone marrow cycles made white blood cells and over-produced the bad one, the Gleevec attacks it and kills the bad one. This caused him to experience regular fevers, muscle pain, and flu-like symptoms every two to three weeks. Using a military metaphor, his wife described the bad cells as a foreign force trying to take over a territory they did not own. "There's literally a war going on," she explained. Despite the side effects of his daily required medication, Donald did not meet the criteria for Social Security disability benefits, which is determined by the stage of the disease and on the drugs that are required for treatment.

For a while, Donald received health insurance through his wife's employer. The first time that his wife went to pick up his prescription for Gleevec at the pharmacy, it was close to $5,000. After this surprise, and each time his wife changed employers or her employer changed to a different insurance company, his wife had to "go through the battle" of getting his medication pre-authorized. The prescribed monthly medications for CML were still expensive, typically costing between $50 and $80 after the pre-authorized insurance coverage.

But at the time of the interview, both Donald and his wife were unemployed, without health insurance, and were having difficulty finding jobs. Donald was looking for a new oncologist while navigating the medical world without health insurance, a confusing and stressful endeavor. For the time being, Donald was eligible for free medication, but he and his wife also faced a financial barrier to routine medical tests because of their lack of insurance.

Concerns over job security were expressed by some who worked at Whirlpool and who were confronting the possibility of choosing between the health or financial security of their families. Additionally, job security and longevity were impacted by the need for parents to take extended time off from work, a recurring theme among parents, while supporting their sick children. Concern about their financial futures added to their economic burden. One man stated, "I'm very nervous about one of us losing our jobs. . . . I mean, everything would be gone. We can't afford it on a less paying job. We can barely afford it now, especially over the years you get behind with charged things on credit cards, you know gas to go to the hospital, you start jackin' up credit card bills."

Among other factors, financial difficulties are more commonly seen among young or older patients who lack social support, have dependent children, and have low income or little savings. In the absence of social safety nets, families had to adjust to their financial struggles. Participants used their savings, relied on family and friends for financial help, or made changes to household spending that resulted for many in a reduced lifestyle.

The Hiseys, who had built their home, did end up making the difficult decision to sell it to downsize and pay off debt from medical bills. While seeing their old bedroom lights on in their former home when they drove by at night was hurtful for everyone, the family acknowledged that not being so tight on bills took the pressure off everybody.

THE FUNDRAISERS

"Nobody does fundraisers better than Clyde." This is something I would hear repeatedly during my fieldwork. More than a dozen articles or advertisements for fundraisers or memorial events appeared in the local paper, the *Clyde Enterprise*, during my first year of fieldwork. From chicken or spaghetti dinners to auctions, bake sales, memorial runs, Little League baseball games, and golf outings, fundraising efforts for affected families occurred regularly. Some memorial fundraisers, which occur annually, no longer need a description of whom they represent because their histories are well known and have been absorbed by the community.

Fundraising efforts have seeped into the physical environment of the community as well. Tip jars for donations decorate gas station and restaurant checkout counters. Solicitation for support funds continue to appear at bars, fairs, sporting events, and even the cafeteria at the high school. Cancer awareness stickers adorn cars. Cancer centers and radiation treatment facilities that are peppered throughout the town, including a Cleveland Clinic Cancer Center adjacent to Whirlpool (see Figure 4), have been described as simultaneously "weird but convenient."

Businesses themselves are philanthropic, and items, including food, for these events are often donated from companies around the area. The Second Annual 5K Run/Walk for Bubba held in 2014, for example, included a pancake breakfast for which Croghan Bank donated napkins, Gary's Diner donated pancake mix, and Whirlpool donated sausage. In June 2018, I took my own son to a fundraiser held at the high school for a young boy with cancer. We purchased tickets for "carnival" game stations set up in the gymnasium. A mascot for the local fire department was another feature of the event, as well as a dinner.

In contending with social anxieties about cancer, institutions adapted and evolved as part of the coping process. The local schools have also participated in a system that has evolved in the community in response to the cancer cluster with nurses actively engaging in the care and reintegration of sick children. Parents, physicians, and school nurses have become more vigilant to signs of illness. Nurses offer guidance to other students so that they know how to treat an ill

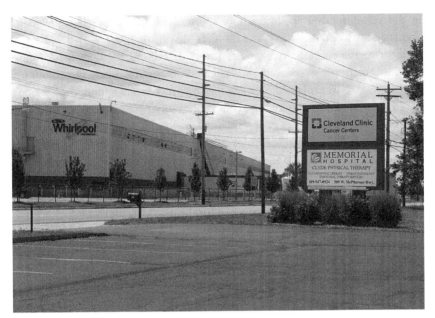

FIGURE 4. Image of a Cleveland Clinic Cancer Center adjacent to Whirlpool Corporation in Clyde, Ohio, Sandusky County. (Photograph by Laura Hart.)

child returning to school and how to limit germs, and they prepare students for the fact that sick children coming back to school might look different but still need friends. One resident described an event—"cancer week"—where, each day of the week, elementary students wore a different-colored ribbon representing a different type of cancer. Children are initiated into the culture of community by wearing hats and ribbons to school to support sick children. A grandmother shared the story of her granddaughter whose entire kindergarten class wore hats each day so that another classmate who lost his hair from treatment would be more comfortable. At the end of the year, her granddaughter donated her own hair to go toward kids like him.

In the small town of Clyde where everyone was "connected to each other," it was difficult not to know somebody impacted by cancer, and in that sense, fundraisers have redefined what it means to be a part of the community. In one way, the repeated interactions at these events function as a means of building shared identities and social relations, providing a measure of unity within the town and drawing residents closer. People take pride in the outpouring of compassion and participation, perceiving those things as normal responses to the emotional impact of a cancer diagnosis. The new collective identity of Clyde has evolved by giving cancer a deeper meaning and has broadened the significance of what it means to be a Clyde resident. As one resident, Barb, explained, "there is a lot of good support for the sports, but we have just as much or more for the fundraisers."

In this sense, fundraisers, like school sports, have themselves become social events on the weekends—a type of resource-sharing that is necessary for being a member of the community. Some residents describe these appeals for funds, which occur nearly every weekend, as being unique identifiers of community affiliation. As Carl explained, "It's like if ya haven't been to a fundraiser or don't have a wristband, then you're not in our community."

Community fundraisers gave residents a way to be proactively involved and helped buffer the financial hardships that victims faced. The town became very efficient at hosting fundraisers, raising significant amounts of money for affected families. Those who did not have a lot to give often volunteered. Turnout for these events was high, with events sometimes even selling out. "Sometimes you want to get a ticket, but you have to wait for the next one," Betty said.

The family of Bubba Andrews recalled that his fundraiser was particularly large. They estimated that 2,500 people attended it and raised $60,000 for their family when Bubba was going through treatment. "There were people showing up to volunteer that I have never even seen before," his brother recalled. Even athletic teams from outside the community came to show their support, and some even wore their own handmade "Bubba's Battle t-shirts." Their family, like other families for whom fundraisers were organized, were very appreciative of the community's support. They discussed how they still see people wearing the t-shirts and bracelets in honor of Bubba. Bubba's mother mentioned her own collection of t-shirts she had acquired from fundraising efforts. With two drawers of "nothing but fundraising cancer t-shirts," she proudly wore them to work every day. She recited them for me: "Bubba's Battle," "Taylor Tackles AML," "Alicia's Army," "Scotty's Smokehouse," "Team-up for Tanner," "Hugs for Alexa." Shirts with messages often promoted the child as a superhero or soldier standing up against the threat of disease. She recalled that she was wearing Taylor's shirt to work on what happened to be the day she died.

The more intimate relations within the community result in people feeling a sense of responsibility to each other. Therefore, as reflected in the collective fundraising activities, they participate in this sharing of resources. Despite the positive outcomes of fundraising and the community, some acknowledged the contradiction in this unique community attribute. Why was fundraising necessary to begin with?

Not only were people made sick by the likely inaction of the state in protecting community health, but those in need and dealing with illness were often left to navigate care with underfunded health care systems and inadequate financial support. Echoing the constraints placed on families by state welfarism, Carl reflected, "I mean it's just like everybody knows what to do and how to make it a success, but that's pretty sad when you think about it." As the state abdicates its responsibility for protecting citizens, solutions must then be self-realized as community members try to counterweight the hardships experienced by families. Offsetting the unequal financial burden is itself a form of social welfarism, as the community, on a small scale, assumes the responsibilities of the state without its structural means of support. This type of philanthropy is inevitable.

This sharing of resources—albeit impressive and positive—redistributes the unfair burden in a particularly capitalist way. In its endorsement of a mode of individualism, it dulls a sharper political critique reflected, in part, in the lack of support for families as they searched for the environmental source of contamination. Families impacted by disease struggled alone for many years to get the information they needed from the state health departments and Environmental Protection Agency (EPA) after being told that there was likely an environmental link to the cancer cluster. The broader community was especially unsupportive of the lawsuit against Whirlpool. Despite poor community turnout at the first public informational session held by the lawyers since the filing of the lawsuit, impacted families made their pleas for community support. Sierra Hisey, whose childhood was largely defined by watching both her brother and sister battle leukemia for years as they went through treatments, was just eleven years old at this meeting when she spoke to the adults dispersed across the bleachers. Standing in the large gymnasium holding an oversized microphone alongside her father, she seemed remarkably small and stood out among the other when she said, "You do not want this to happen to your family."

On the one hand, the generosity offered by the community was recalled positively by participants as a demonstration of their compassion for the impacted families. Yet some recipients received judgment and criticism from within the community, especially after the filing of the lawsuit. The fundraisers were an expression of charity that helped cement social solidarity in the community. In receiving funds, though, there was a sense that the families were, in turn, obligated to a sort of unspoken contract related to the maintenance of those social relationships. The filing of the lawsuit against Whirlpool and the decision to move from the community were perceived as violations to that contract. In this sense, this system of mutual accounting, as Derrida describes it, is itself a kind of economy infused with economic rationale.[16]

But charity and the potential compensation from the lawsuit were linked to ideas about worthiness. "Well, I know a few in it for the money," one resident observed. Families were sensitive about this. Conveying awareness of ideologies about morality and work ethic, Donald frequently assured me that despite his illness, "work-wise, I'm kind of very strong work ethics and very strong morals." Dave felt pressure to keep his opinions about the cancer cluster to himself due to the reaction of his friends and the implied condemnation coming from the community regarding the legitimacy of his family's financial need.

We have a pretty nice house, but we built it ourselves. We did all the work ourselves and we worked hard. We have both worked the same job for twenty-nine years, and I manage the grocery store. A lot of people think I own it, but I don't, I just manage it for somebody. You have these fundraisers to help try to pay for bills and to keep life normal for the kids, and sometimes you feel like people are questioning why you need that. "You could sell your house." We heard that, you know. Well, everything else has been taken away from the kids, you know, their friends . . . so we were gonna do whatever we could to keep the house. And, you know, so you have these fundraisers you help make the house payment 'cause your wife's off work for two and a half years through it all, and we get people looking at us. Before Tyler got sick we planted the pine trees out there and they were guaranteed. After Tyler got sick, our friends had a fish fry for us and the fire department raised some money. Right after that Perri's Plantation was out here replacing some of the trees that had died that they guaranteed and then some people were saying stuff about how we just had this fundraiser and "they're out buying trees," you know. So it's just . . . it's just uh, I feel it's very stressful.

In the narrowest sense, criticism of how funds were used by recipients reflected suspicion that their motives in accepting donations were deceptive. On a larger scale, charity fraud, when legitimate, affronts the altruistic motives of those who donate thinking they are helping fulfill a need, creating a sense of unity in confronting a problem. But the "strings attached" sentiment directed by some at the Clyde families had no real merit and was demoralizing for recipients. Dave Hisey recalled this feeling of disillusionment when he learned that critics attached his worthiness of receiving help to his income and how he spends his money:

We'd always go to Michigan for vacation and the kids would swim in a lake up there. That was our vacation every year, and you know, the kids really love swimming. So they couldn't swim because Tanner had this port in and there was worry of infection so we started talking about having a pool that if you chlorinate it yourself and don't let other people in, they can do that and it's something enjoyable . . . just family time, you know in the backyard, bonding. So we asked someone about that at Swim Rite Pools and then he calls me back a couple days later and says, "Hey, I talked to a few of our lenders, and they can donate some of the stuff for a pool." And I go, "Oh, that, that's pretty cool." Then they started talking about an in-ground pool, so we ended up getting an in-ground pool. We still had to pay some money, but we cashed in our 401k and paid for it that way. It's something for our family. I mean, at that point we were thinking, we want to spend as much time with them as we can. So you find yourself doing things like that for them but it looks bad to other people if you had a fundraiser. But you wanna create some memories, and you want to give them some fun while you can. It plays mind games with you because. . . . But we did get a pool, and we paid for it, I did a lot of the work myself on it, paid buddies to help, you know, we poured the concrete ourselves.

Some participants noted a culture of resentment toward the few families that chose to move out of Clyde. An example was cited of a family who dealt with their five-year old's diagnosis and death. This family had received financial assistance from the community in the form of fundraisers. While initially supported by many, when the family chose to move from Clyde while their son was sick, Travis, a family friend, recalled that some people turned against them and "badgered them with the question, 'Why did you move?' 'You left us, you left the town, you left the community, we supported you.'" The suggestion of betrayal implicit in comments such as these was again an unstated inference that boundaries were attached to the help received—sharing resources was, in part, about bringing the community together and, as such, moving from the community was a sort of betrayal.

The families of children with cancer also participated in a kind of sharing of resources and building of community, albeit less conditional, as they gained unanticipated insight into some of the specific problems associated with managing illness. Like an heirloom passed on from one family to the next, they shared tips and tricks for helping their children cope. Community building among stricken families occurred as resources were shared and giving acts mitigated the harsher realities they faced together. Dave recalled the thoughtfulness of a gift from the grandfather of Kole Keller, another child who had died of cancer: "I can remember them coming out here and bringing a big basket in that hallway. They had this big basket, and it was just a big fluffy pillow pad. And you could put it on a twin-size bed, and it just makes it more comfortable. We would have never thought about that, but somebody got that for them, they got it for us, ya know, then we got it for somebody else. But it just, you pick up little things that made life easier when we were there."

Dave also recalled that when his daughter was in the hospital for chemo treatments, she stopped talking to people because she was frustrated, scared, and sad. In response to the around-the-clock poking and prodding of nurses, and the beeping backdrop of her hospital room, she closed in on herself and began to respond to questions with "Hm, mmm." So, when Dave's employer bought her a computer, it allowed her to escape into movies and also to communicate with her friends if she wanted to. Having a computer temporarily helped her escape from her sadness and the monotony of the hospital experience and gave her an outlet to the outside world. When Dave's son was also diagnosed with leukemia, with three and a half years of ensuing hospital visits, Dave's family did the same thing for him. Dave said, "You know, I'd spend the night with him up there, and I would come home and he and I would have Rocky Fest, and watch all the Rocky movies. It just let him escape."

The Hiseys then began giving computers to other sick children. Involving his own kids in charitable acts also gave the children a proactive way of countering the negativity of their experiences. There was a twofold benefit to involving his children in acts of giving. On the one hand, it gave a sense of empowerment to his children. On the other hand, it gave other sick children a sense of hope when they saw his children in remission, allowing them to see that they had a chance to be healthy again.

As a childhood cancer survivor, Chase Berger has also become an advocate for other children with cancer. During his senior year of high school in January 2020, he organized a fundraiser for an eleven-year-old fifth grade boy. Chase did not know the boy or his family but learned about his story—that he was battling cancer for the fourth time since being diagnosed at age three. With an initial modest goal of $800, Chase sold the 325 spaghetti dinner tickets at the local VFW within the first thirty minutes of the event, and then began reusing the tickets. His networking and outreach efforts led to an $11,100 benefit for the family. That night, he finally got to meet the boy. Chase recalled this moment: "[This was] all I really cared about. I just wanted to see him smile. Like I just wanted to see the smile on his face and that was really my worry. You know, is he going to smile? You know, he's going through such a hard time. And as soon as we came through the door, there was a big smile on his face. And that was just, really, the biggest thing that hit me, like, 'This is awesome.'"

Chase intends to continue to fundraise for other kids, with a plan to institute an annual grant to high school seniors who have experienced cancer directly or within their family. This, he explained, would help these seniors go on to college.

After Alexa died, the Browns traveled to Washington, D.C., to promote childhood cancer funding. Her parents, Warren and Wendy, also started a foundation, Alexa's Butterflies of Hope, in her honor. The foundation began as a way in which to raise money to help support local families whose children had contracted cancers with the financial cost of transportation, treatments, and hospital stays and has since expanded. By providing a result, fundraising is productive in that it helps to reduce a sense of helplessness and increases the hope that one may overcome difficult situations.

ATTEMPTS TO MANAGE RISK WHILE COPING WITH UNCERTAINTY

Toxic disasters tend to psychologically affect victims more grievously than natural disasters or human-made accidents, as evidence of its existence and its psychological impact on human bodies are frequently invisible. Their origin and impact tend to be opaque, and they are frequently harder to resolve; usually, toxic contamination has no clear endpoint or even a starting point, and that uncertainty is anxiety-inducing.[17] The sinister nature of contamination is also exacerbated by its ongoing nature and the inexact science of remediating the problem. Contaminated communities are often characterized by stress and anxiety as they come to grips with that possibility. This is exacerbated when products and profits are assigned more value than humans and when industry is able to avoid responsibility, making the cause unknown. Not being able to identify the source of risk affects our understanding of it and allows it to proceed without intervention. For those living with embodied risk, environmental risk becomes omnipresent, which not only perpetuates fear but also normalizes it as families routinely navigate their lives in a reality characterized by uncertainty.

While all health risks are similar in some ways, their meaning is shaped by the alleged source of the hazard. In contaminated communities, adverse outcomes may be attributed to toxic exposure even if there is no way to prove the relationship, and this happened to Clyde residents who began to question previous illnesses within their families.[18] In addition to challenging people's paradigms, perception of environmental contaminants affected lifestyle choices wherein people's way of living, relationships, pattern of activities, and places needed to sustain these activities altered to accommodate a changing reality.

Perception of risk also varied across participants based on their experience living with embodied risk. Living with embodied risk, and directly experiencing the impact of cancer on their social identities and lived experiences, brought the possibility of ever-present risk to their consciousness. These families became more aware of cancer and toxins generally, signaling the vulnerability of everyone to disease, including their own risk of cancer and death. Making decisions about how to live offered them some possibility of managing their risk and taking control of their life circumstances. Many attempted to reduce risk in their long-term lived experiences by mobilizing surveillance. Risk reduction required constant management and was still perceived as limited due to the great deal of uncertainty and ambiguity that characterized their lives.

Affected families were often questioned by outsiders as to why they did not simply move. For impacted families, this was a complicated question. Those who had firsthand experience with embodied risk had a more acute awareness of what it meant to be in danger, but this conflicted with their desire to maintain normalcy in the lives of their families. They also wanted to feel a sense of belonging in the community.

In spite of the implied criticism of his parental decision to stay, Dave explained that it was not easy to leave home. He and his family ultimately chose to stay in Clyde because of their jobs and social ties and to keep their children in the school system near friends and support systems. While he and his wife contemplated moving away, they did not definitively know what the source of the cancer was, and they wanted to minimize stress on their family. "You want to do everything to protect your kids, but at that point we didn't really know what we were protecting our kids from," he explained. The benefits of staying in the community were more important.

Wendy and others echoed his response. "If you move fifty miles away, how can you know that it will be a safe place?" she said. Some acknowledged that if they were young and had a child, they would consider moving from Clyde, but ultimately they made no plans to leave. Strong family ties and the attachment to the community, particularly among older, longtime residents, made it difficult for many to move away from Clyde. "We were born and bred here. This is our home," I heard repeatedly. "Moving is unthinkable." Bubba's mother explained: "You love the people. Oh my god, they're your family! Your life is here. It's your life. Your life! It's all I've ever known. . . . I had a reporter come up to me at a benefit and ask me, 'Would you have raised your child anywhere other than Clyde?' and I said, 'Absolutely not.' And they said, 'Why, why would you keep your kids here? Why would you stay here?' And I was like, 'Look around this community. There's not a greater community in this world than Clyde, Ohio. There's not. The community is amazing."

Chase, too, shared this sentiment, expressing that he definitely wanted to raise a family in Clyde. He said, "I just love the city of Clyde too much and the people in the city. You know, that's home. No matter what happens, we all support each other." For many, having a sense of belonging in the community meant having a guiding purpose among others who shared their values.

Not everyone shared the same enthusiasm about raising a family in the community, though. None of Bubba's siblings, for example, expressed the desire to live in or raise children in Clyde, potentially interrupting the established generational continuum of raising families in the community. His youngest brother explained: "I feel like I'm breathing chemicals in, every single time I go back to Clyde. I just feel like I'm breathing in poison and killing myself every time I go back." Another resident, Erika, spoke of her son: "When he got out of the Marine Corps, he moved to Cleveland to go to college and he doesn't wanna raise kids in Clyde because three people in the block [my husband] grew up in, three of the boys that grew up together died within like three to five years of each other of cancers."

Some younger families expressed the desire to move but were concerned that they would not be able to sell their house due to depressed property values created by the cancer cluster designation, an issue Michael Edelstein refers to as the "inversion of home," wherein the meaning of home shifts from a locus of family security to a place of danger and degradation.[19] One's safe, rooted place not only is threatened by contamination but also has material consequences in the financial reversal in home value it creates. Karen felt stressed about the value of her property when, after contacting her bank to inquire about refinancing for a home equity loan, the bank suggested not starting the process of refinancing, implying that the property value may be lower. Michelle added, "I'm really concerned about living here now, but my husband and I can't afford two house payments. Nobody's gonna wanna buy this property now. And the refinancing company is requesting that we have soil testing done because of what's going on next door. And the soil testing is going to come out of our pocket. If they are requesting

PCB testing, that could be twelve to fifteen hundred dollars, and I don't have that to put forth. We just don't know what to do, but we're afraid to stay here."

Although financially unable to relocate, Keith expressed wanting to keep his children from visiting for long periods of time: "I have two young daughters, thirteen and fourteen, from my previous marriage and I'm much more conscious. One of my daughters wanted to come for six weeks this summer. I'm not gonna allow her to come. I don't want her in that environment any more than she is. I'm worried. I'm concerned. They still don't know what it is."

Because of the responsibility assigned to the government to assess and mitigate environmental health risks, it is reasonable to assume it would meet that obligation in responding to the problem. Yet many felt that the state officials dropped the ball with the cancer cluster investigation as they encountered obstacles in accessing health care. This, along with reduced government expenditure on public and social services, created a quagmire scenario which, for many, resulted in a cost prohibitive lack of resolution.

One consequence of weakening traditional institutions intended to safeguard public welfare is that citizens must rely on themselves as self-governing agents, often through modifying their consumer and lifestyle choices. Even though they did not know the exact source of contamination, residents tried to protect themselves from suspected toxins in their homes. They made strategic decisions to protect their families, for example, by having their ponds and wells tested even before the involvement of the EPA and Health Department, by changing their well water to city water, or through the installation of water filtration systems in their homes. Some students at the high school brought bottled water to school to avoid drinking water from the fountain. Families also bought bottled drinking water for their homes to avoid possible well water contamination, put air purifiers in their bedrooms, or made changes in their food choices.

By attempting to minimize their exposure to chemical risk through product selection and through tasks such as grocery shopping and safety improvements in the home, residents became what Dayna Scott refers to as "citizen-consumers."[20] In this framework, the market is the predominant medium through which many families must manage their own exposure to risk. Women and mothers in particular act as consumer gatekeepers for their family's safety from chemicals as these practices are embedded in everyday life.[21] Bubba's sister reflected on how her brother's experience with cancer changed the way that she lived:

The concern for getting cancer and the concern to get healthier has really affected my husband and I. We buy all organic, local produce and meat, we buy organic milk, we drink filtered water, we don't use water bottles, we use the reusable stuff, we don't use paper plates. We've just completely changed our lifestyle in the way that we eat and the things that we do because of that concern. We want to take all of the precaution that we can to make sure that we're doing everything that we can to not get sick. I think that's really hit home for us.

Where fear of risk merges with ideologies surrounding motherhood and responsible living, risk becomes a tool of governance. Companies have lured conscious consumers into being responsible participants in family health care by offering products that look "green." This type of manipulation is productive in the sense that consumer choice makes individuals feel more empowered in protecting themselves and their families. It becomes repressive when those who do not make the "correct choices" are labeled deviant or irresponsible in terms of protecting their families. More generally, as observed by social movement scholars, societal emphasis on lifestyle politics may even deter from more effective collective efforts toward institutional-level, systemic change as individuals channel their social change energy to a micro-level response.[22]

However, with the perception by some Clyde residents that toxins and hazards could be present anywhere, concern was voiced about the pervasive sense of losing control over health and lifestyles. "You can be bombarded with things and you can try to be as safe as you can be in a lot of areas, but you just can't get away from everything," Wendy explained. Finding the balance between managing risk and maintaining normalcy was implicit in comments such as these. There were also financial limits to protecting oneself and one's family when the price of products such as water filtration systems was often cost prohibitive.

Additional concerns were voiced about the safety of homes, gardens, and the actual soil residents lived on. "I'm afraid to dig anything in the soil . . . you know, plant flowers." They expressed regret about losing the ability to have what other people take for granted. There was a level of caution now attached to their daily activities. Concerns about toxic exposure were pervasive. One Whirlpool employee, Erika, expressed having heightened concerns about occupational hazards and often thought about toxin exposure while working:

I always thought about it 'cause once in a while I work up in the department that my girlfriend worked in and I would work overtime. They would clean these things out, and there's all this junk dripping on ya, and they want you to wear these white paper suits and boots and it was hard getting around in 'em because they were real small, so a lot of times none of us wear the boots and it wasn't mandatory, they just said so you don't get your feet all wet because you walk through all these chemicals and stuff, and they're dripping on ya. And they're dripping on your mouth, and your hair, and sometimes I'm thinking, "Why am I doing this?" It's probably why my friend got sick, and that's before the cancer cluster really was brought out or anything. I was doing this and now I'm thinking, "Why did I ever go in those departments? Why wasn't I thinking more about what would go through my skin?" So sometimes, yeah, you're sitting in there and you're working away and you're bored, the factory's monotonous and you think, "Okay, what am I breathing in here?" There's a total mist at the department next to mine. When you look over there, it's like a mist—a vapor, all day, every day. . . . They won't let it go out in the air so they've supposedly pumped it back in through a filter into the plant right where we're working. So sometimes it makes you wonder, "What am I breathing in?"

Those in close proximity to Whirlpool Park were also concerned about PCB runoff in their well water. Karen, a mother of two children with developmental delays and cognitive disorders, lamented the fact that their family memories were now tainted with suspicions of toxin exposure. In reflecting on the park, Karen recalled,

People used to envy us because we lived so close to Whirlpool Park—because it was so convenient. It would be so crowded in the summertime so we'd wait until just about dinnertime because we always ate early. My [mother-in-law] always had supper on the table when her husband came in 'cause he farmed, so they had a specific amount of time for him to eat and get back out in the field. So then I just kinda carried that on, and we'd already have our supper ate and we'd go over there by the time everybody was leaving to go home and eat and then it wouldn't be crowded at all [laughs]. It's too bad that your memories are being, you know, tarnished. Because now it's like when I think about when I had my son's birthday party over there, and all my nieces and nephews were over there in the creek gathering up the frogs. . . . I mean you just think, I don't know—were we safe or weren't we?

MANAGING EMBODIED RISK AMID CONCERNS ABOUT THE FUTURE

For most, the impact of the cancer diagnosis did not end with the conclusion of treatment. It involved ongoing participation in medical surveillance, a continual reminder of their body and environment as sources of danger. Because of possible late side effects, childhood cancer survivors need lifelong follow-up care. For some, fear and uncertainty also remained, even after treatment was successfully completed.

Both Tyler and Tanner are in remission but still must deal with ongoing and long-term problems stemming from disease. Tanner takes growth hormone shots every night because he is in the first percentile in growth for children his age, a consequence of having radiation treatment on the pituitary gland. Other participants also stressed the point to me that the experience of illness—whether active or "cured"—affects one's daily life forever. It is not simply something that can be put away at the end of the day.

Chase described living with cataracts and having to wait for the condition to continually worsen before being eligible for laser eye surgery: "I never really thought I would have cataracts. I never would've thought in a million years that my eye would have to be sewn halfway shut like it is because I've never met anyone that has their eye sewn halfway shut. Like, never in a million years would I ever think that, but you know it happens and we just have to deal with it."

Not many people knew about Chase's recurrent doctor checkups and eye problems, but he framed this as his personal battle that, like cancer, he would have to overcome independently. Survivorship and the idea that being positive is a choice were central to his identity.

Donald, the currently unemployed fifty-two-year-old who is in remission from CML, continues to take medication that kills the fats in his bone marrow, resulting in strong flu-like symptoms every two to three weeks. Additionally, because his immune system is compromised, he is more vulnerable to more extreme illness, including bronchitis and pneumonia, than other people. Betty also discussed her daily concerns about her exposure to germs because her immune system is compromised by the removal of her spleen, which regulates infections.

The Hiseys, along with other families, were burdened by concerns about the future. A sense of foreboding infiltrated their everyday lives, along with an understanding that this issue would be protracted and chronic. Some projected that toxin exposure would affect the health of many more families in the future, including their own. "I worry every day. In the restaurant business, I see families every day and I wonder who's next," Travis stated. Within this context, suspicions arose about even minor complaints that their kids could have cancer. "You take your kids or grandkids to the doctor for every little thing," Erika explained. Dave and his wife lived with fear of the possibility that they would outlive their kids and wonder who would take care of them if this happened. A cough from one of their children created stress for families as they constantly worried about their health and safety.

Family members adopted different methods of coping, and some parents and children resorted to counseling and medication to deal with issues of depression related to cancer. Despite the toll that cancer took on their daily lives, families still had to deal with the mundane aspects of existence and did not have the option to defer these responsibilities. Dave explained:

> At some point, you get hardened to it because you realize life still has to go on. . . . There are no right or wrong answers. You find yourself feeling bad for yourself one minute, then you get up, put your pants on the next day and the floor needs swept, you know, the food needs cooked, the yard needs mowed. I mean, life doesn't wait for you. But you just try to live life the best you can and try to do the right things. People might think you're not doing the right thing and you might not be, but I wish some of them could be more understanding of our situation.

Dave's decisions, like those of other parents, were motivated by advocacy for his family and were rooted in his desire to promote stability amid the chaos of his family's experience.

The affected families in the Clyde cancer cluster remained cohesive in this aspect. Their struggles with the unknowable did not alter the integrity of their families. The impact of cancer on their lives put them on the perimeter of a traditional experience of family within the community. As the sphere of responsible parenthood expanded within this cultural context, wherein the source of toxicity was unknown and accountability was impossible to achieve, families without financial resources, time, and stability were pushed further to the margins of what was considered normal. Families were most immediately concerned with managing their everyday lives and were grounded in the needs of their loved ones. The imperative for self-protection created psychosocial and practical conflicts as they adapted to the impacts of cancer on their families and in their community.

ADAPTING TO CANCER AS A WAY OF LIFE

A dissenting faction of the Clyde community emerged after repeated unsuccessful attempts to get the help they needed through traditional means of recourse failed. These impacted families continue to live under the assumption that there is, in fact, great risk present and that no one entity will ever be identified as liable. They made choices to become more proactive in their encounters with risk. Other than choosing to leave Clyde, which few have opted to do, this faction of the community has shifted to a more cautionary model of living. And families who lost children may have had their traditional perception of the community altered by the fact that they were not universally supported. While still engaging with and living under the umbrella of the broader community, this faction shared a certain inchoate sense of group identity, distancing itself from one of the core ideologies of the broader community—that of seeing Clyde as a harmless, idyllic place.

The passage of time would have inevitably transformed Clyde despite the cancer cluster. But because of it, and the attention it drew, changes to the town's identity as a cancer cluster were more immediate. Cancer fundraisers, which became commonplace and continue to be regularly attended, are the most obvious indicators of this adaptation. The course of social action on the part of the broader community stopped there, perhaps because institutional change itself provokes anxieties. The message remains that Clyde is a supportive and giving community. Yet, although the identity of the broader community changed, it was not in ways that addressed the original problem of risk, eliminated the presence of risk, or protected the community from future catastrophe. In the case of Clyde, people have adapted to the consequences of contamination even as cases of cancer among children and adults in the community persist.

5 ▸ TOWARD TRANSFORMATIVE MOVEMENTS OF THEORY AND PRACTICE

The chapters in this book map out the mechanics by which inequality operates in one of many small communities dealing with industrial pollution and elevated levels of cancer. History is important to this mapping because it helps explain how larger social forces affect individual circumstances of members of a society. Neoliberalism is an inherently racialized, gendered, and classed system in that its operation depends on inequality along these social lines and others. The inequalities that surface in response to its imposition on the day-to-day lives of people are context specific. The history and logics of neoliberalism help illuminate connections between the decline of the welfare and regulatory state and its subsequent effects on environmental regulation. But history is also a tool for understanding the structural source of ideologies that we take for granted today—those that serve as a function of subordination. This is important because as ideologies infiltrate culture and daily life, their structural sources—in this case, the individualization of risk and health, and emerging related ideologies such as "post-truth" and anti-science—become difficult to trace.

But merely exposing or deconstructing ideological and historical bases of oppression falls short of a full critique. Insofar as ideologies mean anything, they mean something in everyday life. The most useful space for analysis is where ideological knowledge that governs meets the actual experiences of people. The relationship between people and their agency in determining their life outcomes and the structures that constrain individuals is complicated. Looking at how the dynamics of deregulation coupled with neoliberal logics played out in the actual lives of people in this case study reveals that institutions impose a kind of framework for thinking about and organizing our lives. Identifying contradictions in participants' accounts exposes how people become objects of institutional practices.

Yet "place"—irrespective of complex institutional orders—is also a powerful contributor to the ways in which people interpret their lives. This complicates a framing that understands community responses to suspected environmental contamination as merely a matter of economics—that people will simply choose their jobs over health. Homing in on practices of power—what happens on the ground in conflicts such as this one—reveals three important things. First, othering itself is inherent in the meanings people attach to place. Second, risk is used to reproduce and maintain concepts of selfhood and group membership. And third, emotions play a key role in the reproduction of inequalities. Making these tensions visible also shows how these relations are organized in various material ways.

By and large, the community of Clyde, although threatened by catastrophe and risk, changed to accommodate risk, rather than substantially alter it. An understanding of how this happened points to the repressive and productive capacity of risk. This book has examined different types of risk—environmental risks and risks inherent in social structure (e.g., the economy), risk that is socially produced through the work of emotions, and embodied risk. Each can be distinguished, but the interplay between them reveals that risk is a product of the sociohistorical context and perpetuates the social structure, providing the basis for social reproduction. This framework highlights the dialectic relationship between structure and agency and helps explain how factions of residents are reconstituted through marginalization within their own communities. Four intersecting systems of power worked to hamper a collective sense of community subpolitics in this case study. Each of these domains is grounded in a particular type of risk that places constraint on the community's culture and ideologies and that plays out both on the macro level and in everyday experiences.

ECONOMIC POWER

Reflected in the complexity of risk assessment, profit-motivated definitions (and redefinitions) of risk are imposed by the very institutions that created the problems in the first place. Alongside efforts to enhance human health and happiness, science is increasingly used in the unregulated pursuit of economic gain at the expense of the health and safety of communities.

At the community level, an industry and a community may operate for many years in a mutually beneficial manner, both financially and socially. A community's acceptance of a regulating entity depends to some degree on the belief that the power entrusted to them will work to further the interests of all involved. But when a population becomes more economically dependent on the industry, decisions can be made that threaten the least powerful stakeholders. In this case study, the distribution of economic power in the community made the community economically dependent and, consequently, less likely to engage in activities that would threaten the existing arrangement. As with other communities with a heavy industry presence, financial dependence on the town's largest employer had a direct impact on the community response to risk that many suspected was generated by that same corporation. Financial concerns limited residents' actions, as reflected in residents' complacency with maintaining the status quo and in employees' fear of standing up to a corporation. Workable solutions for protection from environmental hazards are in direct conflict with the threat of personal financial ruin. How does someone select from presented disasters? Does a person decide to move away from contamination, or to lose that person's job? Thus, the economic distribution of power not only positions groups differently within the community but also shapes their resistance, or lack thereof.

The question arises as to what degree of environmental risk is acceptable in a company's enterprise of profitability. Residents of Clyde did not anticipate that their community would be environmentally degraded or that members of the community would become ill, and they did not foresee this as being the price of participation in an economic system from which they also benefit. Yet a percentage of human casualties is the seeming consequence of living within a community characterized by risk. It is not simply that human casualties occur but that they are now considered as probable and acceptable in the pursuit of strategic economic advancement. Although resultant personal tragedies attract public attention to catastrophic events, they are largely unproductive as motivators of system-level change.

INSTITUTIONAL ORGANIZED IRRESPONSIBILITY

Industry and government mutually interact to define, interpret, and manage risk. As evidenced in the case study of Clyde, the inadequacy of government in protecting a community's health is inevitable given the outmoded systems through which risk levels are determined, as well as the increased influence of industry in decision making that has eroded local-, state-, and federal-level interventions. Existing power structures resist acting to retroactively repair harm and eventually cannot do so because problems become so far removed from their scope of management. Rather, they operate within a distortion of order which confuses and misdirects attempts at modification or redress. Borrowing from

Ulrich Beck, the term "organized irresponsibility" implies intentionality, although at some point the dysfunctional elements of unregulated, human-created hazard may appear to have a "life of their own" which is, in fact, no longer subject to intervention or control. Response to these outcomes emerges instead, as coordinated efforts to deflect responsibility, with both industry and government "tossing the ball" to one another as they attempt to avoid accountability for cause or reparation.

STIGMATIZATION

Stigmatization plays multiple roles in the operation of power. First, residents experienced a sense of external stigmatization by its classification as a cancer cluster. The perceived threat to the community's character negatively impacted not only its economic identity but also residents' sense of pride and their perception of Clyde as an unspoiled rural American community. The perception of outsiders mattered to residents, and there existed a sense of exclusivity in the town's quiet, unblemished wholesomeness. Residents were connected through their high level of satisfaction with an existing coherent arrangement that had been successfully spinning for decades. When critical media attention was directed at Clyde, the changing identity of Clyde was met with resistance and a detectable sense of loss and was, perhaps, one of the strongest barriers to a unified response to the contamination issue.

The second way that stigmatization operated within the town was evident in the divisive method used to censure voices threatening the status quo. Criticism of Whirlpool's suspected complicity in the environmental contamination of Clyde was often met with reproach and condemnation, as it was perceived as a threat to the character of the town. Rumors circulated about lawsuit participants, whose motives and methods were questioned. In this regard, emotions did the work of subordinating and isolating plaintiffs and other critics of Whirlpool. While the experience of having a child with cancer placed people on the perimeter of normative parenting to begin with, the larger community contributed to affected families' sense of isolation initially through lack of support and ultimately by not aggressively dealing with the problem of risk. As the once cohesive community splintered, some dissenting voices were further marginalized by efforts to legitimize the broader community's inaction.

NEOLIBERAL INDIVIDUALIZATION

Life in contemporary society is progressively self-directed. This can be seen most evidently in the situation that presented in Clyde, where traditional avenues of recourse to address harm failed. The consequential individualizing logics that influence the perception of environmental risk contribute to its normalization as the tasks of managing risk become more personally determined and are woven into daily life. Environmental risk is further legitimized by its integration into social dialogue through media and public health policies that promote deterrence and avoidance of harm as matters of individual preventive choice. In the case of Clyde, caregiving, family decision-making, and even consumer selections became acts of individualization as affected residents considered their own courses of response to contamination. Measures taken (such as the purchase of bottled water, water filtration systems, etc.) not only empowered residents but qualified their personal investment in the outcome by strategically redirecting responsibility of outcome to the individual. As a result, perceptions of environmental risk influence the experience and response to risk, while at the same time obscuring and legitimizing the operation of other systems of power.

RISK ADAPTATION BEYOND CLYDE

Unfortunately, Clyde is not the only disease cluster in Ohio.[1] Several other suspected disease clusters have been reported since the 1990s. Environmental contaminants and local industries were implicated in the Village of Wellington, Ohio, where residents were found to be 3.7 times more likely to develop multiple sclerosis (MS) than the rest of the country. In Marion County, Ohio, a push by residents to investigate the high cancer rates among graduates of the River Valley schools led to the Ohio Environmental Protection Agency (Ohio EPA) discovery that the high school and middle school were built on a former U.S. Army waste dump where students could have been exposed to more than seventy-five hazardous contaminants. However, the state health department ended the investigation of eighty-three leukemia cases after five years without determining a cause because of a lack of direct evidence that the chemicals caused the cancer. And less than three hours east of Clyde, residents of East Liverpool, Ohio, have been breathing heavy metal–contaminated air for eleven years from a hazardous waste incinerator.

Numerous communities outside Ohio have experienced parallel experiences with illness and suspected chemicals. Struggles for justice in predominantly Black and Hispanic communities dealing with contamination are grounded in a more entrenched history of racial and ethnic disenfranchisement. From the crisis in Somerville, Texas, where residents are contracting stomach cancer at a rate as much as forty to sixty times the national average, to the lead water crisis in Flint, Michigan, that has affected about 100,000 people, institutional racism has played a more insidious role in decision-making processes and in health outcomes in their communities.[2] Using Flint as an example, the arrogant presumption by city officials that they could get away with malfeasance and that the population of Flint had no political power or resources to fight back was rooted in the social determinants of the Flint community. It was not until someone with a "pedigree," in this case a pediatrician who recognized a rising trend in lead levels among Flint's children, raised the alarm that attention was brought to the situation. Even now, despite national outrage, the problem persists as actions to determine accountability for the water crisis stall.

Existing literature on experiences with contamination suggests that environmental risk is experienced differently in racialized communities compared with predominantly white communities. Due to a long history of institutional racism and interpersonal discrimination, racialized communities do not experience the same levels of safety and security as white communities. A world in which whites have been prioritized and where the symbolic meaning system of whiteness has been repeated through generations establishes a different societal norm rooted in the privilege that entails and sits in opposition to expectations of racialized communities. Whereas the status of American citizenry for whites carries with it presumptions of administrative protections built into civil and federal systems of government, racialized communities have low expectations that government will respond to their environmental problems. As found in the case of Flint and other cases, communities of color dealing with human-made crises experience feelings of distrust in public officials.[3]

In addition to being a significant determinant of the health outcomes and expectations for resolution, race impacts response to disaster, with activists of color often viewing community contamination as part of a longer history of racial injustice, and ultimately seeing themselves as connected to the racial justice movement.[4] Differences in social capital and how race affects the lens through which assumptions of risk are viewed might underlie findings that communities of color are more likely than whites to confront polluting industries.[5] Yet contaminated communities of color are less likely to receive media recognition or government support.[6] The lack of media attention might be explained by sociologist Robert Higgens's argument that the social meaning of race is conflated with pollution, and that minority environments are deemed "appropriately polluted spaces."[7] Social pollution practices—those that work to construct the racial "other"—also help to make invisible the disproportionate level of environmental pollution within minority communities. Marginalized neighborhoods tend to be associated with territorial stigma, labeled from both outsiders and insiders as dangerous, run down, and poor.[8]

It is important to consider the assumptions that drive powerful political and social constructs and are implicit to systems of structural advantage (or disadvantage). Presumptions of status exist as a determinant to how environmental risk is addressed and is inherent in our identity as individuals and as part of a group. Presumptions of advantage due to race and ethnicity and other markers of social standing contribute to action and inaction in the face of risk events. Challenges directed at these anticipated norms threaten to deconstruct life patterns and can contribute to schisms within the communal whole, evoking emotion-based responses. This has implications for social change because when decision-making is motivated by emotions such as fear, it can be difficult to see alternative solutions or come up with new ideas. It can also contribute to stereotypes and prejudice as people overlook more relevant information in favor of stereotyped shortcuts to categorize people.[9]

The conflict in Clyde was organized around the establishment of group-based differences, sharing a set of common processes and conditions with other types of conflicts. While expressions of othering are contextual and vary greatly, they contain a similar set of underlying dynamics that suggest that othering is a broader phenomenon. Othering presents in constructions of community and in narratives of personal injury. A close examination of the ways risk discourses operate as strategies of normalization, of exclusion and inclusion, demonstrates the centrality of notions of othering in how people think about and act out risk. In Clyde, the process of exclusionary behavior leveled against the plaintiffs effectively relegated them to a status of other. Themes of fear, otherness, and belonging permeate personal narratives and public texts. They echo those of value and valuelessness that underpin racial politics and other processes of marginalization.

Emotion impacts presumptions of place-based identity and the system under which it operates. Given the certainty that contamination of communities like Clyde will continue, this book provides insight into evaluating community responses that occur in toxic places by assessing residents' perceptions of and responses to risk. But Clyde is just one community, and while the strategic selection of this case makes it well-suited to produce context-dependent knowledge, comparative case studies are necessary to expand our knowledge further. For example, because environmental racism means that racialized and otherwise marginalized communities disproportionately house toxic industries and bear the related health and environmental disparities, it would be interesting to examine how different communities' *expectations* of being toxic impact how emotion works across these cases and how risk is subjectively experienced. Do shame and pride operate differently in these contexts? How does this impact a community's decision to engage, or not, in collective action? In Clyde, although there was no racial divide between Whirlpool's defenders and the all-white litigants, the process of exclusionary behavior was leveled against the plaintiffs, effectively relegating them to a status of other. Are scripts around fear, othering, and belonging universal? Who gets othered in a racialized community, and how do its members navigate moral orders imposed upon them? How do racial identities affect embodied risk? Where racialized communities become home to devalued polluting industries, what lies beneath the meanings their residents attach to "community" to drive or hamper collective action? And to what degree does racial discrimination intensify the effects of exposure to physical chemical agents?

Emotions and other embodied experiences can help us understand civic responses to environmental issues.[10] Recognizing emotion-laden narrative techniques of various stakeholders can expose dynamics of stigmatization and deeply held values that often define intergroup conflicts. Becoming more aware of how emotion contributes to residents' perceptions of contamination might lead to the identification of general discursive and institutional patterns, and new ideas for how to interrupt them.

WHERE POST-TRUTH MEETS ENVIRONMENTAL SCIENCE

An understanding of emotions, subjectivity, and identity is critical as fear, anxiety, grievances, and anger increasingly feed into various genres of right populism, with implications for science and the environment. The relations between public science and private profit have shifted significantly over the past fifty years with a broad national and global movement toward neoliberal policies. Social welfare–oriented organizations have been marginalized in the United States and internationally, with the neoliberal network's efforts to discredit the authority of the United Nations (UN) and other social welfare–oriented agencies while simultaneously advancing neoliberal economic policies. While the G8 is the center of power of the "transnational state," the International Chamber of Commerce (ICC) works to advance international policies in line with the neoliberal agenda.[11] There is also evidence that regulation is increasingly taking place in international governance bodies, which has simultaneously led to deregulation in some areas (such as the reduction of national trade barriers) as well as pressures for stronger international standards for the production, storage, and distribution of internationally traded goods.[12] The influence of transnational corporations—and their backing by industrial science—has also increased, subordinating international institutions to their wider agendas. Neoliberal reforms can now be imposed outside of standard political channels by supranational organizations.

By the time Donald Trump and the 115th Congress took office in 2016, the political-economic forces of neoliberalism had already established themselves as part of a regime of scientific management. Prior to the Trump administration, some in the scientific community had already expressed concern about a "war on science" and the rise of populist antagonism to the influence of experts.[13] This came to fruition when the Trump administration launched federal environmental policy into an unprecedented era of environmental deregulation, making vast changes to U.S. environmental policy and limiting federal funding for science and the environment.

The administration's actions related to climate change were the most highly profiled. President Trump signed an executive order dismantling Obama-era climate actions, including the Environmental Protection Agency's (EPA) Clean Power Plan, which was designed to reduce carbon dioxide emissions from new and existing power plants.[14] Shortly thereafter, Trump announced that he would pull the United States out of the Paris Agreement, a global collaborative agreement with 194 other countries to curb planet-warming greenhouse gas emissions.

In February 2017, President Trump signed a joint resolution passed by Congress revoking the U.S. Department of the Interior's "Stream Protection Rule," which had placed stricter limits on dumping mining waste into surrounding waterways.[15] As the former head of the U.S. EPA, Scott Pruitt—a figure who, in his prior role as Oklahoma's attorney general, frequently sued the EPA over its regulations—quickly dismantled the EPA's power in favor of industry and economic growth. Under Pruitt's direction, the EPA withdrew an Obama EPA request that aimed to better track the industry's methane and volatile organic compound (VOC) emissions by obtaining detailed information on oil and natural gas facilities.[16]

The administration also changed the way pollutants are regulated. Countering the advice of the EPA's chemical safety experts, Pruitt rejected a petition requesting that the EPA ban all use of chlorpyrifos, a pesticide that has been shown to be associated with brain damage in children and farm workers, even at low exposures.[17] Pruitt's "back-to-basics" agenda promised to clear the backlog of new chemicals awaiting EPA approval. After heavy lobbying by the chemical industry, the EPA also narrowed the scope of its risk evaluations by changing the way the federal government determines health and safety risks associated with potentially toxic chemicals. The EPA excluded from consideration potential exposure from the chemicals' presence in the air, ground, or water. Instead, it would focus narrowly on possible harm caused by direct contact with a chemical in the workplace or elsewhere.[18] While the Trump EPA ended or diluted new rules that never went into effect, chemical industry lobbying and campaign donations effectively defeated legislation aimed at regulating chemicals, including per- and polyfluoroalkyl substances (PFAS), a group of human-made fluorinated chemicals that do not break down, accumulate over time, and are persistent in the environment and the human body.[19]

Alongside legislation aimed at deregulation, and in an effort to delegitimize climate science in particular, U.S. government websites were altered to modify or remove their web content regarding climate change. The EPA's Office of Science and Technology removed the word "science" from its mission statement, replacing it with language that instead emphasized "economically and technologically achievable performance standards." In April 2017, an official for the Interior Department, which works under the direction of the U.S. Geological Survey to "help resource managers cope with a changing climate," deleted much of its content on climate change.[20] The EPA similarly scrubbed its explanation of climate change on its website, replacing "climate change" with vague terms such as "resiliency."[21] The EPA dismissed several scientists from an advisory board that reviews the research of EPA scientists, explaining the decision in terms of broadening the diversity of the board to include industry representatives. Additionally, Pruitt proposed allowing the EPA to reconsider making the underlying data for scientific studies publicly available.[22]

The Trump-era EPA was weak in its enforcement of environmental laws to correct noncompliance and promote cleanup of contaminated sites.[23] Lack of priority in terms of environmental law enforcement was further reinforced by deep cuts to U.S. science and environmental agencies, along with environmental programs that protect air and water. In addition to suspending studies of health risks to residents who live near mountaintop removal coal mine sites in the Appalachian Mountains, the White House also ended NASA's Carbon Monitoring System.[24] The EPA also announced changes to the organization of the National Center for Environmental Research (NCER), an EPA group that funds research on children's health and environmental health disparities affecting minorities and the poor. This raised concerns that the administration was compromising the issuing of grants to outside environmental health researchers and programs that examine the effect of pollution on children's health. Though Pruitt was forced to resign after several ethics scandals, his legacy of active deregulation continued through his replacement, former coal lobbyist Andrew Wheeler.

When the Trump administration's term ended, its key environmental officials rejoined lobbying firms and other pro-industry think tanks. The Biden administration made moves to repeal Trump-era regulations that weakened the government's ability to protect public health, but industry remains actively involved, influencing environmental policy. Lobbying and campaign donation spending from top chemical manufacturers are expected to remain high in opposition to industry-opposed restriction.[25] Several members of the EPA's Science Advisory Committee on Chemicals, which conducts peer reviews of chemical risk evaluations, are employed by companies with direct financial interest in specific chemicals or by consulting firms hired by those companies to represent their interests. Industries have played a role in the development of cancer guidelines and health assessments for chemicals such as arsenic, vinyl chloride (VC), butadiene, and dioxin.[26] Scientists employed by or affiliated with the chemical industry continue to serve on advisory committees that evaluate the health risk posed by an industrial chemical and other scientific review panels. And the neoliberal ideology that has made these actions possible continues to infuse right-wing populist movements, parties, and figures whose aims are to reverse the trend toward big government and state intervention while at the same time defending the "ordinary people" against an allegedly "corrupt elite." Promoting broad brush attacks on the government, embodied in the phrases "drain the swamp" and the "deep state," helps advance the idea that government is bad and is in service to deregulation and the private market.

Environmental researchers have long been familiar with the type of misinformation campaigns that have become more commonplace today in the "post-truth" era, as assaults on scientific integrity and science-based policy have historically presented in communities dealing with contamination. The case of Clyde also reveals the workings of a parallel dynamic—that risks can be used to regulate human behavior and the threat of unknown risks can be used to push people toward political agendas. Appeals to emotions and personal belief are key to shaping public opinion.

It remains to be seen how this heightened era of post-truth—the dismissal of science, evidence, facts, and truth itself—will affect environmental policy in the long term. Endemic to contemporary populism, post-truth reflects the populist strategy of valorizing common sense over expertise. As Tuukka Ylä-Anttila observes, though, it also involves the advancement of politically charged alternative knowledge.[27] The creation and communication of counter-knowledge serves as a mobilizing function for social movements by creating epistemic communities to counter those of the establishment and construct new identities.[28] This is why leaders associated with post-truth discourse demonstrate their contempt for the establishment so publicly. Counter-knowledge requires a different knowledge orientation—one that professes belief in truth to be achievable by alternative inquiry. In some ways, post-truth is characteristic of the obfuscating tactics used by industry and to the benefit of the economic elite. But it also creates a crisis for neoliberal governance, which has relied on offering the public a narrative of nonpartisan expertise and objectivity in policy to be perceived as credible. Perhaps this crisis is reflected in the fact that the share of Americans with confidence that scientists act in the public interest has actually increased since 2016, with slightly over half saying they trust scientific research findings more when the data are openly available to the public and when the research is not funded by an industry group.[29] This is also reflected in the massive mobilization against the recent right-wing administrations in the United States and United Kingdom, and growing environmental movements across the globe.[30] As history has shown us time and again, politically volatile moments also hold potential for being pivotal ones.

RECULTIVATING THE PUBLIC SPHERE

Part of what it means to be in a community is to have a common set of goals, practices, and values that allow people to continually weave their meanings and practices into a shared social fabric. Communities are sacred to democracy, as they are a setting wherein strong democracy can present—where public discussions and debates can take place and the concerns of private citizens on the one hand are mediated against state interests on the other. If communities are held together, in part, by their ability to come together around agreements based on the practical effects of certain issues, then their failure can have dire consequences. Several factors today undermine deliberative democracy. For example, Jürgen Habermas observes that although economic fluctuations and downturns are intrinsic to capitalism, public perception of such potential crises is that they are the result of ineffective governance and a disjointed response from the state.[31] With its increasing reliance on scientific knowledge to forecast and control economies, citizens have lost not only faith in the state but also their belief in rationality. This, in turn, has reduced the levels of meaning and motivation felt by citizens.

Further, once we create governing institutions, these same institutions come to limit how we think about new problems and how we communicate with each other.[32] We tend to think of only solutions that exist within the confines of the rational systems we create, often deferring to private market approaches over humanistic policies. This explains why, for example, the United States has over half of a million people who are homeless and why thirteen million children experience food insecurity.[33] It reveals how despite our country's great wealth, tens of millions of Americans cannot obtain basic health care and why health care is not viewed as a right that should be made available to everyone, but rather as an economic good. It also helps explain why, in Clyde, when many children and adults began presenting with disease, economic arguments trumped the ability to reason based on human values. It illustrates how the various institutions we create influence and stifle the way we think about new problems so that we are no longer thinking freely, and we begin to advance governing systems ahead of our lives and communities. Such efficiency-first thought has changed our value structure in that as people become increasingly individualized, they lose their sense of responsibility to one another.

Alongside policies that reward industrial activity is a cultural aspiration to wealth that prevails in the United States and elsewhere. The addictive quality of consumerism reaches across all demographics, propelled by hundreds of messages suggesting that a good life is attainable by working hard, making money and spending it on products that claim to make us happy, loved, esteemed, and perhaps a sense of belonging. This has come at a high price for the well-being of both people and the planet. Research consistently shows that the more that people value materialistic goals, the lower their subjective well-being and the higher their depression and anxiety.[34] Strong materialistic values also influence our social relationships, with people less likely to act empathetically in generous and cooperative ways. And when people are under the dominion of materialism, concern for the environment tends to diminish.[35]

The possibility of consensus and reasonable action is dependent on the degree to which democratic communication about risk can be achieved. To resolve disagreements about risk, our exchanges must be free of ideology. What this means in practice today is that it is imperative to elucidate the roots of crisis—to critically investigate how perceptions of risk are influenced by processes that transcend the political realm. As Thomas Scheff observes, in a culture where people learn to act independent of others, there is also a tendency to hide emotions. One outcome of this suppression, in Scheff's words, is that "emotion vocabularies in modern languages are ambiguous and misleading, so that they tend to hide alienation."[36] Ahmed reminds us, too, that what is relegated to the margins is often "right at the center of thought itself."[37] With the tendency for forms of domination to actively obscure historical and contemporary forms of inequality, reading emotion where it is assumed to be irrelevant can make visible the state of our relationships.

Not only does neoliberal capitalism foreclose robust social and environmental legislation in the public interest, but our current phase of capitalism is inimical to democratic communication.[38] Exposing the distortions, misrepresentations, and political values found in our knowledge and speech is therefore important for recultivating our democracy and our humanistic values.

Ethnographers have an important opportunity in this area, as they can closely examine verbal accounts, gestures, and contextual details to help make visible the role of emotion as a mechanism of power. Because ideas and strategies around risk often operate at the symbolic and conceptual level, researchers can and should read the work of emotions when they are unnamed and should make sense of logics that work outside the immediate consciousness and overt articulation of their practitioners.[39] To the advantage of ethnographers and interviewers doing this investigative work, the everyday language of emotion is based on the presumption of interiority. Although people are often aware of which emotion is socially appropriate, the sociality of emotion likely remains unconscious for most people. As such, the disparity between participants' conscious reflections and their subconscious dispositions is not methodologically limited. Evaluating what emotions do in ethnographic case studies may bring us close to explaining what people do with words and deed.

Citizens more generally need to become familiar with the patterns of risk discourses employed to reach specific outcomes, often with a consequence of reproducing inequalities, so that they become part of our repertoire of knowledge. This is increasingly important in a politically polarized society where emotionally charged dialogue around race, class, and gender is strategically used by governments to dampen activists' power. As people increasingly turn to social media as a news source, recognizing the affective basis of risk perception should be taught as a media literacy skill. While social media can facilitate the mobilization of the public toward important civic issues, it also hinders the quality of discourse happening in the public sphere, and public debate has become fragmented. In addition, with no clear solution to the problem of fake news, which spreads more often than accurate stories because of the emotion it provokes, the need for media literacy is essential for our democracy. Nothing could reinforce the importance of this more than the public opinion control efforts of China, which has one of the most sophisticated censorship regimes in the world. Most recently, China has begun a campaign for greater state control under the banner of "positive energy," a program geared toward regulating public opinion through the promotion of content that provokes happy feelings.[40]

Like all skills, the ability to critically interpret distortions and misrepresentations and to identify political values is realized through practice. Because science, health, and risk are shaped by political and economic relationships that are not value-neutral, activists play a key role in educating and empowering disenfranchised communities. The Center for Health and Environmental Justice (CHEJ), a nonprofit environmental group established by environmental activist Lois Gibbs, is an example of one such group that is helping threatened communities and working to keep intact constitutionally guaranteed freedoms. Some of this work involves creating spaces for democratic public dialogue and informing citizens of their rights and civic responsibilities. At public hearings about environmental issues, for example, residents are often told by officials that they cannot speak, with the implication that they are illegitimate sources of knowledge. This exclusion of the presence and experience of subjectivities not only is inherent in the work of creating authority but is a threat to democratic communication and contributes to distrust, as across the board, people want to trust that elected officials will act in the interest of the people.[41] CHEJ works to reinforce conditions of equity, education, and balance in community discourse in part by providing neutral venues for public exchange.

While science remains an important tool for environmental activists, science alone will not improve communities. In Gibbs's words, science is comparable to "a screwdriver, but not a hammer."[42] There are not always laws that activists can wrap their hands around because the policies in place are often written by the companies themselves. And government environmental policy itself is often limited in scope. This is reflected in cost-benefit analyses that literally assign monetary value to human lives and weigh this against the costs of contamination cleanup. Environmental permits may even specify the acceptable number of human deaths permissible per air pollutant from hazardous waste incinerators. Through laws and court decisions, state institutions organize and enforce the environmental politics of everyday life, assigning human value that renders relations of inequality normative. Laws and legal decisions (such as *Citizens United v. Federal Election Commission*) that bestow personhood status to corporations contribute to this imbalance by affirming corporate overreach into political decision making. Because such implemented laws and legal decisions are often designed to protect industry interests at the expense of people's well-being, the only way to change these dynamics is through demanding political power. Community activists can help residents work "outside the box" as they develop tactics to stop threats to their community. This requires looking at positive alternatives that connect to real local needs. When communities struggle in their efforts to develop a cohesive plan, as often occurs, advocates can offer their assistance.

Messaging becomes another important facet of this advocacy because it directly relates to getting people involved. A short, accessible, positive message conveys the purpose of the community group and encourages people to join in the cause. Advocates at CHEJ, for example, reinforce the importance of saying "no" to particular damaging actions in a community while identifying a message to which they are saying "yes." Rather than affirming broad goals such as renewable energy and conservation, these messages are grounded in the community's local needs and convey a specific action.

One recurrent government and industry talking point in contaminated communities, which are often in economically depressed areas, is the emphasis on retaining jobs or bringing more jobs to the community. The case of Richmond, North Carolina, a primarily low-income African American community, provides an example of how to use that narrative to the benefit of local activists. There, where the community was rallying against mega dumps, staff at CHEJ held a town meeting to help residents develop an economic plan. Residents came together to discuss what it was that their rural community did not have that they needed, citing ideas such as a movie theater and social services. Using the Chamber of Commerce's own language, they made a case for building alternative jobs and presented it to the state senator and local government officials. As a result of their self-advocacy, some of their suggestions were implemented. When capital is place-bound, the community has a higher degree of control over it and can better assert their interests.[43] A key source of empowerment for burdened communities is to establish agency through proactive rather than reactive means. This type of citizen engagement helps divorce the idea of "good citizenship" from neoliberal self-governance. New achievements based on pragmatic dialogue can increase the levels of meaning and motivation felt by citizens. Enthusiasm surrounding democratic projects can also generate attention from and engagement with the broader public, serving as a catalyst for new social justice initiatives.

With their trove of experience, grassroots leaders are most effective at pragmatically transforming communities. Activists are not constrained by disciplinary boundaries and are intimately connected to challenges faced by large numbers of ordinary people which can, in turn, help them develop innovative insights and achieve a better impact for their research. Academic scholars and policy makers across the disciplines can play an important role in assisting grassroots efforts, offering rigorous research and frameworks to study the interaction between social organizations, demographic problems, and technological issues toward the goals of developing effective governance institutions and living peacefully with the environment.

Several legislative efforts to further improve regulation are occurring. Short of federal legislation that would shift the burden of proof onto "those who create the hazard, benefit from the hazard, or advocate for the hazard," some state legislators have passed bills to identify and communicate the potential for hazardous chemical exposures which could be harmful to human health, particularly to vulnerable or susceptible populations, such as children and pregnant women.[44]

In the summer of 2022, CHEJ announced its "Unequal Response, Unequal Protection" campaign. CHEJ presents a model that resolves the problem of the Agency for Toxic Substances and Disease Registry's (ATSDR) inability to adequately determine the safety of people in an affected area due to limits with risk assessment. When ATSDR is called upon by the EPA or a health department to conduct a public health assessment at a Superfund site or other location with suspected disease-causing chemicals, its task is to quantify risk. But ATSDR relies on data collected by the EPA, which is always incomplete, as the EPA does not conduct exhaustive testing of an entire area. As Jose Aguayo, a senior scientist associate at CHEJ, pointedly observed in my interview with him, ATSDR must extrapolate from the data that it has available, and this is not conducive to its task of determining whether people are living in an affected area. Further, he noted, "traditional methods of risk typically occur within a lab setting wherein researchers have full control of the exposure and other variables, but risk assessment does not translate well in a dynamic environment where control of the different variables is lost." In collaboration with community leaders and scientists, including an epidemiologist who studied environmental contamination at the U.S. Marine Corps Base Camp Lejeune, North Carolina, CHEJ designed an alternative approach to evaluating health problems in communities—one that identifies potential chemical health hazards based on Presumptive Association. This approach mirrors the process used by the U.S. government when considering adverse health effects suffered by veterans, active military, first responders, 9/11 victims, and others exposed to toxic chemicals. As in the case of Camp Lejeune, where water was found to be contaminated with industrial solvents, benzene, and other chemicals from the 1950s through the 1980s, the U.S. Department of Veterans Affairs (VA) established a presumptive service connection for potentially exposed veterans, reservists, and National Guard members who later developed one of eight diseases for which there is scientific evidence to support the creation of presumptions. The government also used a presumptive approach to justify disability compensation policy for Vietnam War veterans potentially exposed to Agent Orange. Nearly 19.5 million gallons of herbicides, some of which contained dioxin, were sprayed over Vietnam between 1961 and 1971 by U.S. military forces during the conflict.[45] In the absence of limited relevant science and poor exposure data, the VA established a "presumptive" or automatic service connection between potential exposures and the health problems suffered by those veterans. This recognition led to the government providing health care, treatment, compensation, and other assistance needed due to exposure to toxic substances suffered while serving our country.[46] In communities where people have been exposed to toxic chemicals through no fault of their own, CHEJ details a model where the government would extend a similar application of the presumptive approach. Importantly, each step of the proposed investigation process would be bound by a timeline and would be community-driven, involving the formation of a Community Leadership Team (CLT) and an independent Presumptive Review Board (PRB). The CLT would be the decision-making body that drives the health investigation, and the ATSDR response team would coordinate its assembly and aid the CLT in moving through the steps in the investigation. The PRB would be composed of an independent committee of scientists who would use the Presumptive Association approach to analyze the chemicals present in the community and the health effects seen.

While the push for policy reform at the federal level remains important, state and local policy can have large effects on day-to-day life for many people. Evidence-based policymaking is important at the state and local levels. Yet at the state and local levels, change is made easier because, in contrast with the federal government, which is required to do extensive analysis of the rules and regulations it makes, state and local governments face fewer bureaucratic barriers. Different jurisdictions have made different assessments of the problems they face, leading to policies that are specific to their locality. At the same time, state reform efforts may even hold potential for becoming models of national reform. One example of this is Hawaii's model for health-care reform. Hawaii's program is based on an employer mandate that requires employers to pay at least 50 percent of the cost for any employees who work at least twenty hours per week for four consecutive weeks, and it has been successful in restraining health-care costs.

State and local governments also enact laws and regulations that define how economic activity takes place, including environmental regulations, and play a crucial role in ensuring that the public is protected from environmental damages. As another example, California's Proposition 65 (Prop 65) requires businesses to provide warnings to Californians about significant exposures to chemicals that cause cancer, birth defects, or other reproductive harm.[47] The list of chemicals is updated each year and now has about 900 toxins and carcinogens on it. Although federal agencies like the Food and Drug Administration and the EPA already set levels for safe consumption of chemicals, Prop 65 goes above and beyond federal standards, sometimes setting different limits. While Prop 65 has been criticized for equalizing risk in its labeling of all chemicals, some of which are considered low risk, the legislation has led companies to remove or reduce potentially harmful chemicals from their products. The law has also been key in ensuring accountability among manufacturers and retailers whose products contain potentially harmful chemicals.

While the adoption of information and risk-based approaches to mitigating exposures to toxics is important, it still falls short of hazard-based regulatory controls. The narrow focus on precautionary consumption, with its emphasis on individualized strategies based on consumer preferences, is falsely premised on a clear separation and a fixed boundary between the physical body and the natural environment. It is misguided in its presumption that individuals can control the movement of toxics between the environment and the body. Material feminist theorists take the view that boundaries between nature/culture and environment/body are permeable and mutable.[48] Such a reframing expands the kinds of political and ethical interventions that can be made from merely individual efforts to keep toxics "out."[49] A reevaluation of our relationship to the environment—not only our bodies but other ways of living that are ecocentric and sustainable—is also important.

Although this element of his work has been somewhat neglected by environmental scholars in favor of a focus on environmental social movements, Émile Durkheim offers a sophisticated understanding of the relationship between environment and society, types of solidarity, and the division of labor in society. In *The Division of Labor in Society*, Durkheim sees an interrelationship between the physical environment, the size of the population that lives in this physical environment, the technology that is used in the environment, the division of labor, and the type of social solidarity of the community.[50] Each of these components interacts with each other and constitutes a system akin to what environmental researchers today would call an ecosystem. This is a productive way for social scientists and grassroots organizers to think about problems of the environment. It resonates with new environmental movements geared toward the development of healthier environments. One such movement is the degrowth movement. Recognizing ecological problems in the context of a longer historical trajectory of the world economy as a system driven by capital accumulation, its advocates are pushing for a shift from GDP growth of the economy toward more efficient improvements and sustaining ecosystems. Other policy ideas include changing how money is produced and circulated, shortening the working week, limiting the advertisement of products, regulating the planned obsolescence of products, and redistributing wealth.

Similarly, bioregionalism, a movement based on the idea that human activity should be largely restricted to distinct ecological and geographical regions to promote sustainability, imagines a restructuring of regions with a mindfulness toward local environments. Developing deep relationships and practices of care for the environment in specific places not only is necessary for cultivating sustainability but also offers an alternative to neoliberal dynamics of displacement.

We can expect that environmental problems will continue to affect people's ability to reproduce their lives, leading to disruptions such as migration, cultural shifts, increased transmission of disease, and even wars. Climate change is accelerating, which will inevitably lead to pervasive new disputes about risk governance in a growing range of communities.[51] Times of crises, which interrupt our social lives and are marked by periods of uncertainty and change, compel people to adapt to new cultural practices and lifestyles. We saw, on the one hand, how the COVID-19 pandemic revealed cracks in systems of national and global governance with its negative consequences and many still grappling with its health and social complications. Still, the pandemic has had a degree of positive impact on different aspects of lifestyle behaviors. Some of these include more flexible approaches to work, a more localized production and consumption of goods, and a search for many to fill their lives with more meaningful activities. When crises disrupt our social routines and when our social networks are reconfigured, individuals tend to be more open to new ideas and worldviews. Although the next crisis may be different or more destructive, it could provide openings for new configurations of communities and policies that prioritize healthier environments.

Humans are united in their desire to live in healthy communities and have the capacity to innovatively collaborate toward the democratic enactment of policies that are ecologically viable. Improving the well-being of communities involves prioritizing basic needs and reducing inequality. There are important affinities between the vision of a healthy community and deliberative democracy, as public health models tend to bring everyone to the table. As we think about what it means to live well, we must take practical approaches to questions of economic and social injustice, staying grounded in the actual experiences of people. Here, we are also reminded of Patricia Hill Collins, who would ask us, which form of knowing is more likely to lead to social justice—one that denies ethical and moral accountability or one that demands it?

During my last visit in Clyde, I met with the Hiseys at McDonald's. Since my last meeting with them, they had moved from their home of seventeen years to downsize. Now they were closer to the heart of Clyde. Their personal and social relationships in the community were important. "We like being here," Donna explained. They reflected on their experiences, some of which Dave acknowledged they "just want to forget," and talked about their lives since the withdrawal of the lawsuit. Donna has a chronic cough, but the doctors don't know what it is. And still, when Tanner doesn't feel good, he and his family worry that his cancer is back. They wondered if the attention drawn to the company had something to do with the cars downwind from the factory no longer being covered with particles from the burning of chemicals, but they weren't sure. To them, it didn't seem like the community thought much about the cancer cluster anymore and that the broader community had largely settled back into its former civic pattern. They, too, seemed to have accepted that they would not receive justice for their losses. Still, they lightheartedly joked with one another as they talked about the changes in their lives—Tyler's pregnancy, Tanner's experience with community college, and Sierra's plans to pursue a nursing degree. They seemed bonded, a signal of pride in their relationships with one another, and perhaps, too, with the connectedness they felt to their community.

NOTES

PREFACE AND ACKNOWLEDGMENTS

1. Kristina Smith, "'Winesburg, Ohio' at 100," *Ohio Magazine*, December 2019, https://www.ohiomagazine.com/ohio-life/article/winesburg-ohio-at-1001.

INTRODUCTION

1. Warner v. Waste Mgmt., 36 Ohio St. 3d 91 (1988).

2. *Warner*, 36 Ohio St. 3d at 91.

3. "Cleveland, Ohio," Ohio History Central, accessed January 4, 2016, http://www.ohiohistorycentral.org/w/Cleveland,_Ohio.

4. Andrew R. L. Cayton, *Ohio: The History of a People* (Columbus: Ohio State University Press, 2012).

5. "Cleveland, Ohio."

6. "Dow Chemical Company," Ohio History Central, accessed January 4, 2016, http://www.ohiohistorycentral.org/w/Dow_Chemical_Company; "DuPont, Dow Chemical Agree to Merge, Then Break Up into Three Companies," *Wall Street Journal*, updated December 11, 2015, accessed January 4, 2016, http://www.wsj.com/articles/dupont-dow-chemical-agree-to-merge-1449834739; Lucia Fernandez, "Dow—Statistics & Facts," Statista, accessed October 17, 2022, https://www.statista.com/topics/1505/dow-chemical/#topicHeader__wrapper.

7. Basil Meek, *Twentieth Century History of Sandusky County, Ohio and Representative Citizens* (Chicago: Richmond-Arnold, 1909).

8. Meek, *Twentieth Century History*.

9. Dolly Todd Madison Chapter, *Ohio Early State and Local History* (Columbus, OH: Spahr & Glenn, 1915).

10. "From Bicycles to Automobiles," Sandusky County Scrapbook, last updated August 23, 2001, accessed May 26, 2013, http://www.sandusky-county-scrapbook.net/Elmore/Beginning.htm.

11. "Clyde Cutlery," Thaddeus B. Hurd Digital Archive, Clyde Public Library, March 29, 2011, accessed May 21, 2015, http://www.ohiomemory.org/cdm/ref/collection/p15005coll19/id/1470.

12. "Clyde Porcelain Steel Fire, Clyde, Ohio," 1945, Hale's Portrait Studio, Clyde, OH, Thaddeus B. Hurd Digital Archive, Clyde Public Library, September 21, 2010, accessed May 21, 2015, http://www.ohiomemory.org/cdm/ref/collection/p15005coll19/id/1024.

13. SCEDC, "Sandusky County Economic Development Corporation Success Stories," 2014, accessed May 21, 2015, http://www.sanduskycountyedc.net/index.php?page=our-sucess-stories.

14. SCEDC, "Sandusky County Economic Development Corporation Success Stories."

15. "Whirlpool Corporation Recognize Manufacturing Day 2021 by Celebrating U.S. Plant Work Force," Whirlpool Corporation, October 1, 2021, https://www.whirlpoolcorp.com/manufacturing-day-2021-celebrating-us-plant-work-force/; U.S. Census Bureau, "QuickFacts: Clyde City, Ohio," 2021, accessed October 17, 2022, https://www.census.gov/quickfacts/clydecityohio.

16. U.S. Census Bureau, "QuickFacts: Clyde City, Ohio."

17. Phil Brown, "Popular Epidemiology and Toxic Waste Contamination: Lay and Professional Ways of Knowing," *Journal of Health and Social Behavior* 33 (1992): 267–281; J. Stephen Kroll-Smith, and Stephen R. Couch, "What Is a Disaster? An Ecological-Symbolic Approach to Resolving the Definitional Debate," *International Journal of Mass Emergencies and Disasters* 9 (1991): 355–366; Steve Lerner, *Diamond: A Struggle for Environmental Justice in Louisiana's Chemical Corridor* (Cambridge, MA: MIT Press, 2005).

18. Thomas E. Shriver, Sherry Cable, and Dennis Kennedy, "Mining for Conflict and Staking Claims: Contested Illness at the Tar Creek Superfund Site," *Sociological Inquiry* 78, no. 4 (2008): 558–579.

19. Doug McAdam and Hilary Boudet, *Putting Social Movements in Their Place: Explaining Opposition to Energy Projects in the United States, 2000–2005* (Cambridge: Cambridge University Press, 2012).

20. Peter C. Little, "Another Angle on Pollution Experience: Toward an Anthropology of the Emotional Ecology of Risk Mitigation," *Ethos* 40, no. 4 (2012): 431–452.

21. See Kari Marie Norgaard, *Living in Denial: Climate Change, Emotions, and Everyday Life* (Cambridge, MA: MIT Press, 2011); Steven Yearley, *Cultures of Environmentalism: Empirical Studies in Environmental Sociology* (Basingstoke: Palgrave Macmillan, 2005).

22. P. L. Berger and T. Luckmann, *The Social Construction of Reality: A Treatise in the Sociology of Knowledge* (Garden City, NY: Anchor Books, 1966); Mary Douglas, *Risk and Blame: Essays in Cultural Theory* (London: Routledge, 1992).

23. Emily Huddart Kennedy and Josée Johnston, "If You Love the Environment, Why Don't You Do Something to Save It? Bringing Culture into Environmental Analysis," *Sociological Perspectives* 62, no. 5 (2019): 593–602.

24. David Pellow, *What Is Critical Environmental Justice?* (Cambridge: Polity Press, 2018).

25. Carlo C. Jaeger, Ortwin Renn, Eugene A. Rosa, and Thomas Webler, *Risk, Uncertainty, and Rational Action* (London: Earthscan, 2001).

26. R. G. Altman, R. Morello-Frosch, J. G. Brody, R. Rudel, P. Brown, and M. Averick, "Pollution Comes Home and Gets Personal: Women's Experience of Household Chemical Exposure," *Journal of Health & Social Behavior* 49, no. 4 (2008): 417–435; Phil Brown, *Toxic Exposures* (New York: Columbia University Press, 2007); Monica J. Casper, *Synthetic Planet: Chemicals, Politics, and Hazards of Modern Day Life* (New York: Routledge, 2003); Stephen Zavestoski, Phil Brown, and Sabrina McCormick, "Gender, Embodiment, and Disease: Environmental Breast Cancer Activists' Challenges to Science, the Biomedical Model, and Policy," *Science as Culture* 13 (2004): 563–586; Sabrina McCormick, Phil Brown, and Stephen Zavestoski, "The Personal Is Scientific, the Scientific Is Political: The Public Paradigm of the Environmental Breast Cancer Movement," *Sociological Forum* 18 (2003): 545–576; Steven J. Picou and Duane A. Gill, "The *Exxon Valdez* Oil Spill and Chronic Psychological Stress," *American Fisheries Society Symposium* 18 (1996): 879–893; Michael Edelstein, *Contaminated Communities: The Social and Psychological Impacts of Residential Toxic Exposure* (Boulder, CO: Westview, 1988); Kai Erikson, *A New Species of Trouble: The Human Experience of Modern Disasters* (New York: W. W. Norton, 1994); Robert D. Bullard, *Dumping in Dixie: Race, Class, and Environmental Quality* (Boulder, CO: Westview, 1990).

27. S. A. Malin, *The Price of Nuclear Power: Uranium Communities and Environmental Justice* (New Brunswick, NJ: Rutgers University Press, 2015); Noel Healy, Jennie C. Stephens, and Stephanie A. Malin, "Embodied Energy Injustices: Unveiling and Politicizing the Transboundary Harms of Fossil Fuel Extractivism and Fossil Fuel Supply Chains," *Energy Research & Social Science* 48 (2019): 219–234.

28. M. Douglas, *Risk and Blame: Essays in Cultural Theory* (London: Routledge, 1992).

29. Douglas, *Risk and Blame*, 58.

30. See Zygmunt Bauman, *Modernity and Ambivalence* (Ithaca, NY: Cornell University Press, 1991).

31. K. E. Paulsen, "Making Character Concrete: Empirical Strategies for Studying Place Distinction," *City & Community* 3, no. 3 (2004): 243–262.

32. Stephen J. Taylor and Robert Bogdan, *Introduction to Qualitative Research Methods: A Guidebook and Resource* (New York: Wiley, 1998).

33. Kathy Charmaz, "Qualitative Interviewing and Grounded Theory Analysis," in *Handbook of Interview Research*, ed. Dans J. F. Gubrium and J. A. Holstein (Thousand Oaks, CA: Sage, 2002), 675–694.

34. I. E. Seidman, *Interviewing as Qualitative Research: A Guide for Researchers in Education and the Social Sciences* (New York: Teachers College Press, 2006), 79.

35. See Norah A. MacKendrick, "Media Framing of Body Burdens: Precautionary Consumption and the Individualization of Risk," *Sociological Inquiry* 80, no. 1 (2010): 126–149; Rebecca Gasior Altman, Rachel Morello-Frosch, Julia Green Brody, Ruthann Rudel, Phil Brown, and Mara Averick, "Pollution Comes Home and Gets Personal: Women's Experience of Household Chemical Exposure," *Journal of Health and Social Behavior* 49, no. 4 (2008): 417–435.

36. See Kai Erikson, *A New Species of Trouble: The Human Experience of Modern Disasters* (New York: W. W. Norton, 1994).

CHAPTER 1   THE DEREGULATION OF TOXIC CHEMICALS

1. Dieter Plehwe, "Introduction," in *The Road from Mont Pelerin: The Making of the Neoliberal Thought Collective*, ed. Philip Mirowsi and Dieter Plehwe (Cambridge, MA: Harvard University Press, 2009): 1–42.

2. William Robinson, *A Theory of Global Capitalism: Production, Class, and State in a Transnational World* (Baltimore: Johns Hopkins University Press, 2004), 39.

3. David Harvey, *A Brief History of Neoliberalism* (Oxford: Oxford University Press, 2005).

4. Harvey, *Brief History of Neoliberalism*.

5. Kelly Moore, Daniel Lee Kleinman, David Hess, and Scott Frickel, "Science and Neoliberal Globalization: A Political Sociological Approach," *Theory and Society* 40 (2001): 505–532.

6. William Easterly, "Freedom versus Collectivism in Foreign Aid," in *Economic Freedom of the World: 2006 Annual Report* (Vancouver, BC: The Fraser Institute, 2006), https://www.fraserinstitute.org/sites/default/files/EconomicFreedomoftheWorld2006.pdf.

7. Rebecca Lave, Philip Mirowski, and Samuel Randalls, "Introduction: STS and Neoliberal Science," *Social Studies of Science* 40, no. 5 (2010): 659–675.

8. Lave, Mirowski, and Randalls, "Introduction."

9. Lave, Mirowski, and Randalls, "Introduction," 663; Milton Friedman, *Capitalism and Freedom* (Chicago: University of Chicago Press, 1962), 20.

10. Jackie Smith, *Social Movements for Global Democracy* (Baltimore: Johns Hopkins University Press, 2008).

11. DuPont, "1915 Pierre S. du Pont," accessed October 13, 2015, http://www.dupont.com/corporate-functions/our-company/dupont-history.html; Chemical Heritage Foundation, "Henry Herbert Dow 1866–1930," 2017, http://www.chemheritage.org/discover/online-resources/chemistry-in-history/themes/electrochemistry/dow.aspx.

12. Edmund P. Russell III, "'Speaking of Annihilation': Mobilizing for War against Human and Insect Enemies, 1914–1945," *Journal of American History* 82 (1996):1505–1529.

13. Heather Rogers, *Gone Tomorrow: The Hidden Life of Garbage* (New York: New Press, 2006).

14. Advertisement for Du Pont Cellophane from the *Saturday Evening Post*, 1955, dpads_1803 00400, E. I. du Pont de Nemours & Company Advertising Department Records (Accession 1803), Manuscripts and Archives Department, Hagley Museum and Library, Wilmington, DE.

15. "News from Du Pont," display ad in *New York Times*, January 9, 1961.

16. National Academies of Sciences, Engineering, and Medicine, "Industrial Environmental Performance Metrics: Challenges and Opportunities" (Washington, DC: National Academies Press, 1999).

17. D. Kenwin Harris, "Health Problems in the Manufacture and Use of Plastics," *British Journal of Industrial Medicine* 10 (1953): 255–267.

18. V. K. Rowe, Letter to Director of Department of Industrial Hygiene and Toxicology, B. F. Goodrich Company, May 12 1959, http://www.pbs.org/tradesecrets/program/vinyl.html.; Henry P. Smyth, Jr., Inter-company Correspondence, Union Carbide Company, letter dated November 24, 1964, http://www.pbs.org/tradesecrets/program/vinyl.html.

19. The Pesticide Residues Amendment of 1954, Pub. L. No. 83–518, ch. 559, 68 Stat. 511 [codified at 21 USC § 346a (1981)]; the Food Additives Amendments of 1958, Pub. L. No. 85–529, ch. 4.72, Stat. 1785 [codified at 21 USC § 348 (1981)]; Color Additive Amendments of 1960, Pub. L. No. 86–618, 74 Stat. 397.

20. Wallace F. Janssen, "The Story of Laws behind the Labels," *FDA Consumer*, 1981, http://www.fda.gov/AboutFDA/WhatWeDo/History/Overviews/ucm056044.htm.

21. William J. Darby, "Silence, Miss Carson," *Chemical & Engineering News* 40, no.1 (1962): 62–63.

22. *Testimony of Assistant Administrator Office of Chemical Safety and Pollution Prevention (EPA) before the Subcommittee on Commerce, Trade, and Consumer Protection Committee on Energy and Commerce U.S. House of Representatives*, 111th Cong. (2010) (Testimony of Steve Owens, Assistant Administrator, Office of Chemical Safety and Pollution Prevention, U.S. Environmental Protection Agency).

23. Regulations Related to Labor, 29 CFR § 1910.1200-Hazard Communication.

24. Regulations Related to Labor, 29 CFR § 1910.1200-Hazard Communication.

25. Environmental Protection Agency, "Toxic Substances Control Act Inventory Representation for Products Containing Two or More Substances: Formulated and Statutory Mixtures," 2017, https://www.epa.gov/sites/production/files/2015-05/documents/mixtures.pdf.

26. Government Patent Policy Act of 1980, Pub. L. No. 96–517, 94 Stat. 3015 (Bayh-Dole Act, 1980).

27. See Laura M. Brockway and Leo T. Furcht, "Conflicts of Interest in Biomedical Research—the FASEB Guidelines," *The FASEB Journal* 20, no. 14 (2006): 2435–2438; Wayne Kondro, "Conflicts Cause FDA to Review Advisory Committees," *Canadian Medical Association Journal* 175 (2006): 23–24.

28. Food and Water Watch, "Public Research, Private Gain: Corporate Influence over University Agricultural Research" (Washington, DC: Food and Water Watch, 2012).

29. Jon P. Devine, "Has There Been a Corporate Takeover of EPA Science?," *Risk Policy Report* 8 (2006): 35–38.

30. Rebecca Lave, Philip Mirowski, and Samuel Randalls, "Introduction: STS and Neoliberal Science," *Social Studies of Science* 40, no. 5 (2010): 659–675.

31. Lave, Mirowski, and Randalls, "Introduction."

32. Lave, Mirowski, and Randalls, "Introduction."

33. James Thomas, Jill Walker, and Rebecca Westra, "Chemical Trade Prospers in the 1980s," *Monthly Labor Review*, Bureau of Labor Statistics, U.S. Department of Labor, 1991.

34. American Chemistry Council, "U.S. Chemicals Trade by the Numbers," 2020, accessed April 29, 2021, https://www.americanchemistry.com/Policy/Trade/US-Chemicals-Trade-by-the-Numbers.pdf.

35. United Nations Environment Programme, "The Evolving Chemicals Economy: Status and Trends Relevant for Sustainability: Global Chemicals Outlook II Part I," United Nations, 2019.

36. Lucía Fernández, "Revenue of the Global Chemical Industry 2005–2021," Statista, 2022, https://www.statista.com/statistics/302081/revenue-of-global-chemical-industry/.

37. Rebecca Lave and Sara Wylie, eds., "The EPA under Siege," Environmental Data & Governance Initiative, 2017, accessed October 11, 2018, https://100days.envirodatagov.org/index.html.

38. Richard Nixon, "Remarks on Signing the Clean Air Amendments of 1970," online by Gerhard Peters and John T. Woolley, The American Presidency Project, https://www.presidency.ucsb.edu/node/240828.

39. Lave and Wylie, "EPA under Siege."

40. Sarah A. Vogel and Jody A. Roberts, "Why the Toxic Substances Control Act Needs an Overhaul, and How to Strengthen Oversight of Chemicals in the Interim," *Health Affairs* 30 (2011): 898–905.

41. Jordyn Johnson, "30 Years Later, Minden Residents Still Fighting to Clean Up Their Town," *Charleston Gazette-Mail*, June 8, 2019, https://www.wvgazettemail.com/news/30-years-later-minden-residents-still-fighting-to-clean-up-their-town/article_dfdc9df8-6831-59e4-a2f8-432ccbe1ada1.html.

42. Dorceta E. Taylor, *Toxic Communities: Environmental Racism, Industrial Pollution, and Residential Mobility* (New York: New York University Press, 2014); Robert Bullard, *Dumping in Dixie: Race, Class, and Environmental Quality* (Boulder, CO: Westview, 2000); Sherry Cable, Donald W. Hastings, and Tamara L. Mix, "Different Voices, Different Venues: Environmental Racism Claims by Activists, Researchers, and Lawyers," *Human Ecology Review* (2002): 26–42; Sheila Foster, "Race(ial) Matters: The Quest for Environmental Justice Review Essay," 20 *Ecology Law Quarterly* 721 (1993); Paul Mohai and Bunyan Bryant, "Race, Poverty & the Distribution of Environmental Hazards: Reviewing the Evidence," *Race, Poverty & the Environment* 2, no. 3/4 (1991): 3–27.

43. Lylla Younes, Ava Kofman, Al Shaw, and Lisa Song, "Poison in the Air," ProPublica, November 2, 2021, https://www.propublica.org/article/toxmap-poison-in-the-air.

44. J. J. Graff, N. Sathiakumar, M. Macaluso, G. Maldonado, R. Matthews, and E. Delzell, "Chemical Exposures in the Synthetic Rubber Industry and Lymphohematopoietic Cancer Mortality," *Journal of Occupational and Environmental Medicine* 47, no. 9 (September 2005): 916–932; R. S. Luippold, K. A. Mundt, L. D. Dell, and T. Birk, "Low-Level Hexavalent Chromium Exposure and Rate of Mortality among U.S. Chromate Production Employees," *Journal of Occupational and Environmental Medicine* 47, no. 4 (2005): 381–385.

45. Sandra Steingraber, *Living Downstream: An Ecologist's Personal Investigation of Cancer and the Environment* (Cambridge, MA: Da Capo, 2010); Graff, Sathiakumar, Macaluso, Maldonado, Matthews, and Delzell, "Chemical Exposures"; R. S. Luippold, K. A. Mundt, L. D. Dell, and T. Birk, "Low-Level Hexavalent Chromium Exposure and Rate of Mortality among U.S. Chromate Production Employees," *Journal of Occupational and Environmental Medicine* 47, no. 4 (April 2005): 381–385; Sandra Steingraber, *Living Downstream: An Ecologist's Personal Investigation of Cancer and the Environment* (Cambridge, MA: Da Capo, 2010); Michael C. R. Alavanja, Dale P. Sandler, Charles F. Lynch, Charles Knott, Jay H. Lubin, Robert Tarone, Kent Thomas, M. Dosemeci, J. Barker, J. A. Hoppin, and A. Blair, "Cancer Incidence in the Agricultural Health Study," *Scandinavian Journal of Work and Environment* 31 (2005): 39–45.

46. Joanne S. Colt and Aaron Blair, "Parental Occupational Exposures and Risk of Childhood Cancer," *Environmental Health Perspective* 106, no. 3 (1998): 909–925.

47. Colt and Blair, "Parental Occupational Exposures."

48. Grand River Conservation Authority, "Studies Take a Look at Groundwater Quality," *Watershed Report*, 2006, accessed October 9, 2015, www.grandriver.ca.

49. Miquel Porta, "Persistent Organic Pollutants and the Burden of Diabetes," *Lancet* 368 (August 12, 2006): 558–559; World Health Organization, *Environment and Health Risks: A Review of the Influence and Effects of Social Inequalities* (Copenhagen: World Health Organization, 2010).

50. Steingraber, *Living Downstream*.

51. Environmental Protection Agency, *Air Quality Index: A Guide to Air Quality and Your Health* (Research Triangle Park, NC: EPA, 2009).

52. World Health Organization, "WHO's Ambient Air Pollution Database-Update 2014," 2014, http://www.who.int/phe/health_topics/outdoorair/databases/cities/en/.

53. Zoë Schlanger, "EPA Causes Massive Spill of Mining Waste Water in Colorado, Turns Animas River Bright Orange," *Newsweek*, August 7, 2015, http://www.newsweek.com/epa-causes-massive-colorado-spill-1-million-gallons-mining-waste-turns-river-361019.

54. Environmental Protection Agency, "Joint Federal/State Action Taken to Relocate Times Beach Residents," 1983, accessed April 2, 2012, http://www.epa.gov/aboutepa/history/topics/times/02.html.

55. Janet Raloff, "The Pesticide Shuffle," *Science News* 149 (1996): 174–175.

56. World Integrated Trade Solution, "United States Asbestos Exports by Country in 2019," 2019, accessed January 5, 2022, https://wits.worldbank.org/trade/comtrade/en/country/USA/year/2019/tradeflow/Exports/partner/ALL/product/252400.

57. P. Gottesfeld, G. Kuepouo, S. Tetsopgang, and K. Durand, "Lead Concentrations in Labeling of New Paint in Cameroon," *Journal of Occupational and Environmental Hygiene* 10, no. 5 (2013): 243–249.

58. Ohio Department of Natural Resources Division of Oil & Gas Resources, Ohio Oil & Gas Well Locator, 2015, accessed October 8, 2015, http://oilandgas.ohiodnr.gov/well-information/oil-gas-well-locator.

59. Lipophilic chemicals are those that have a tendency to dissolve in fat-like solvents. Begoña Botella, Jorge Crespo, Ana Rivas, Isabel Cerrillo, Maria Fátima Olea-Serrano, and Nicolás Olea, "Exposure of Women to Organochlorine Pesticides in Southern Spain," *Environmental Research* 96 (2004): 34–40.

60. Richard E. Berhman and A. Stith Butler, *Preterm Birth: Causes, Consequences, and Prevention*, report from the Institute of Medicine's Committee on Understanding Premature Birth and Assuring Healthy Outcome (Washington, DC: National Academies Press, 2006).; Jong-Han Leem, Brian M. Kaplan, Youn K. Shim, Hana R. Pohl, Carol A. Gotway, Stevan M. Bullard, J. Felix Rogers, Melissa M. Smith, and Carolyn A. Tylenda, "Exposure to Air Pollutants during Pregnancy and Preterm Delivery," *Environmental Health Perspectives* 114, no. 6 (2006): 905–910; Ligita Maroziene and Regina Grazuleviciene, "Maternal Exposure to Low-level Air Pollution and Pregnancy Outcomes: A Population-based Study," *Environmental Health* 1 (2002): 1–13.

61. Christopher H. Hurst, Barbara Abbott, Judith E. Schmid, and Linda S. Birnbaum, "2,3,7,8-Tetrachlorodibenzo-p-dioxin (TCDD) Disrupt Early Morphogenetic Events that Form the Lower Reproductive Tract in Female Rat Fetuses," *Toxicological Sciences* 65 (2002): 87–98.

62. I. Del Rio Gomez and L. E. Campaigns, *Gender and Environmental Chemicals* (London: Women's Environmental Network, 2007).

63. Guomao Zheng, Erika Schreder, Jennifer C. Dempsey, Nancy Uding, Valeri Chu, Gabriel Andres, Sheela Sathyanarayana, and Amina Salamova, "Per- and Polyfluoroalkyl Substances (PFAS) in Breast Milk: Concerning Trends for Current-Use PFAS," *Environmental Science and Technology* 55, no. 11 (2021): 7510–7520.

64. Ruthann A. Rudel, Suzanne E. Fenton, Janet M. Ackerman, Susan Y. Euling, and Susan L. Makris, "Environmental Exposures and Mammary Gland Development: State of the Science, Public Health Implications, and Research Recommendations," *Environmental Health Perspectives* 119, no. 8 (2011): 1053–1061.

65. Rudel, Fenton, Ackerman, Euling, and Makris, "Environmental Exposures and Mammary Gland Development: State of the Science, Public Health Implications, and Research Recommendations," *Environmental Health Perspectives* 119, no. 8 (2011): 1053–1061.

66. Greta R. Bunin, "Nongenetic Causes of Childhood Cancers: Evidence from International Variation, Time Trends, and Risk Factor Studies," *Toxicology and Applied Pharmacology* 199 (2004): 91–103.; C. A. Stiller and D. M. Parkin, "Geographic and Ethnic Variations in the Incidence of Childhood Cancer," *British Medical Bulletin* 52 (1996): 682–703.

67. American Cancer Society, "Key Statistics for Childhood Cancers," 2021, https://www.cancer.org/cancer/cancer-in-children/key-statistics.html.

68. N. Howlader, A. M. Noone M. Krapcho, D. Miller, A. Brest, M. Yu, J. Ruhl, Z. Tatalovich, A. Mariotto, D. R. Lewis, H. S. Chen, E. J. Feuer, and K. A. Cronin, eds., *SEER Cancer Statistics Review, 1975–2018* (Bethesda, MD: National Cancer Institute), https://seer.cancer.gov/csr/1975_2018/, based on November 2020 SEER data submission, posted to the SEER website, April 2021.

69. American Cancer Society, *Cancer Facts and Figures 2014*, http://www.cancer.org/Research/CancerFactsFigures/index.

70. American Cancer Society, *Cancer Facts and Figures 2018*, https://www.cancer.org/content/dam/cancer-org/research/cancer-facts-and-statistics/annual-cancer-facts-and-figures/2018/cancer-facts-and-figures-2018.pdf.

71. I-Jen Pan, Julie L. Daniels, and Kangmin Zhu, "Poverty and Childhood Cancer Incidence in the United States," *Cancer Causes Control* 21 (2010): 1139–1145.

72. Philip J. Landrigan and Lynn R. Goldman, "Children's Vulnerability to Toxic Chemicals: A Challenge and Opportunity to Strengthen Health and Environmental Policy," *Health Affairs* 30 (2011): 842–850.

73. Landrigan and Goldman, "Children's Vulnerability."

74. John Wargo, *Our Children's Toxic Legacy: How Science and Law Fail to Protect Us from Pesticides* (New Haven, CT: Yale University Press, 1998).

75. Wargo, *Our Children's Toxic Legacy*.

76. Wargo, *Our Children's Toxic Legacy*, 176.

77. An endocrine disruptor is defined as a chemical agent that interferes with the synthesis, secretion, transport, binding, action, or elimination of natural hormones in the body. Sandra Steingraber, *The Falling Age of Puberty in U.S. Girls: What We Know, What We Need to Know* (San Francisco, CA: Breast Cancer Fund, 2007).

78. Steingraber, *Falling Age of Puberty*.

79. Elizabeth Grossman, "The U.S. Government Is Pressuring Europe to Dial Back Its Pesticide Rules," *Mother Jones*, March 17, 2015, http://www.motherjones.com/environment/2015/03/europe-pesticides-endocrine-disruptors.

80. Grossman, "U.S. Government Is Pressuring Europe"; Grand View Research, *Crop Protection Chemicals Market Size, Share & Trends Analysis Report by Product (Herbicides, Fungicides, Insecticides, Biopesticides), by Application, by Region, and Segment Forecasts, 2020–2027*, 2020, https://www.grandviewresearch.com/industry-analysis/crop-protection-chemicals-market.

81. National Cancer Institute, "Cancer Clusters Fact Sheet," U.S. Department of Health and Human Services, National Institutes of Health, 2014, http://www.cancer.gov/about-cancer/causes-prevention/risk/substances/cancer-clusters-fact-sheet.

82. National Cancer Institute, "Cancer Clusters Fact Sheet."

83. Tony Dutzik and Jeremiah Baumann, "Health Tracking & Disease Clusters," *The Lack of Data on Chronic Disease Incidence and Its Impact on Cluster Investigations*, U.S. PIRG Education Fund, September 2002.

84. Dutzik and Baumann, "Health Tracking & Disease Clusters."

85. National Cancer Institute, "Cancer Clusters Fact Sheet."

86. Agency for Toxic Substances & Disease Registry (ATSDR), "Exposure Evaluation: Evaluating Exposure Pathways," ATSDR, 2005, http://www.atsdr.cdc.gov/HAC/PHAManual /ch6.html.

87. Michael J. Thun and Thomas Sinks, "Understanding Cancer Clusters," *CA: A Cancer Journal for Clinicians* 54 (2004): 273–280.

88. Thun and Sinks, "Understanding Cancer Clusters."

89. Wargo, *Our Children's Toxic Legacy.*

90. Wargo, *Our Children's Toxic Legacy*, 173.

91. Wargo, *Our Children's Toxic Legacy*, 173.

92. Robert Goyer, "Issue Paper on the Human Health Effects of Metals," submitted to the U.S. EPA Risk Assessment Forum, 2004.

93. Nelta Edwards, "An Ounce of Precaution," *Contexts* 7, no. 20 (2008): 26–30.

94. The term "citizens" is seemingly used in environmental health studies to invoke the spirit of democratic processes, or often the lack thereof, when environmental and health decisions are made. Phil Brown, "Qualitative Methods in Environmental Health Research," *Environmental Health Perspectives* 111, no. 14 (2003): 1789–1798.

95. Brown, "Qualitative Methods in Environmental Health Research."

96. Fabrizio Cantelli, Naonori Kodate, and Kristian Krieger, "Questioning World Risk Society: Three Challenges for Research on the Governance of Uncertainty," *Global Policy*, Durham University School of Government and International Affairs, May 9, 2010, https://www .globalpolicyjournal.com/articles/health-and-social-policy/questioning-world-risk-society -three-challenges-research-governanc.

97. Cantelli, Kodate, and Krieger, "Questioning World Risk Society.

98. Louise Fortmann, *Participatory Research in Conservation and Rural Livelihoods: Doing Science Together* (New York: Wiley Blackwell, 2008).

99. Michel Foucault, "Governmentality," in *The Foucault Effect: Studies in Governmentality*, ed. Graham Burchell, Colin Gordon, and Peter Miller (Chicago: University of Chicago Press, 1991), 87–104.; Michel Foucault, *Power/Knowledge: Selected Essays and Other Writings 1972–1977* (Sussex: Harvester, 1980).

100. Norah Mackendrick, "More Work for Mother: Chemical Body Burdens as a Maternal Responsibility," *Gender & Society* 28, no. 5 (2014): 705–728.

101. Rebecca Kukla, "The Ethics and Cultural Politics of Reproductive Risk Warnings: A Case Study of California's Proposition 65," *Health, Risk & Society* 12 (2010): 323–334.

102. Kukla, "Ethics and Cultural Politics."

103. Miranda Waggoner, "Motherhood Preconceived: The Emergence of the Preconception Health and Health Care Initiative," *Journal of Health Politics, Policy and Law* 38 (2013): 345–371.

104. Waggoner, "Motherhood Preconceived."

105. Mitchell Dean, *Governmentality: Power and Rule in Modern Society* (London: Sage, 1999).

106. Michael Maniates, "Individualization: Plant a Tree, Buy a Bike, Save the World?," in *Confronting Consumption*, ed. T. Princen, K. Conca, and M. Maniates (Cambridge, MA: MIT Press, 2002), 43–66.

107. Phil Brown, Stephen M. Zavestoski, Sabrina McCormick, Joshua Mandelbaum, and Theo Luebke, "Print Media Coverage of Environmental Causation of Breast Cancer," *Sociol-*

ogy of Health & Illness 23, no. 6 (2001): 747–775; Sandra Steingraber, *Living Downstream: An Ecologist's Personal Investigation of Cancer and the Environment* (Cambridge, MA: Da Capo, 2010).

108. Institute of Medicine Committee for the Study of the Future of Public Health, *The Future of Public Health* (Washington, DC: National Academies Press, 1988), https://www.ncbi.nlm.nih.gov/books/NBK218224/.

109. Elizabeth T. Fontham, Michael J. Thun, Elizabeth Ward, Alan J. Balch, John Oliver L. Delancey, and Jonathan Samet, "American Cancer Society Perspectives on Environmental Factors and Cancer," *CA: A Cancer Journal for Clinicians* 59 (2009): 6.

110. National Institutes of Health, "Arsenic," National Institute of Environmental Health Sciences, 2015, accessed January 7, 2016, https://www.niehs.nih.gov/health/topics/agents/arsenic/index.cfm.

111. National Institute of Health, 2012. "Dioxins," National Institute of Environmental Health Sciences, 2012, accessed January 7, 2016, http://www.niehs.nih.gov/health/topics/agents/dioxins/index.cfm.

112. Ana V. Diez-Roux, "Bringing Context Back into Epidemiology: Variables and Fallacies in Multilevel Analysis," *American Journal of Public Health* 88, no. 2 (1998): 216–222.

113. Diez-Roux, "Bringing Context Back into Epidemiology."

114. Nancy Krieger, "Theories for Social Epidemiology in the 21st Century: An Ecosocial Perspective," *International Journal of Epidemiology* 30 (2001): 668–677.

115. American Cancer Society, *Cancer Facts & Figures 2021*, 2021, https://www.cancer.org/content/dam/cancer-org/research/cancer-facts-and-statistics/annual-cancer-facts-and-figures/2021/cancer-facts-and-figures-2021.pdf.

116. Brown et al., "Print Media Coverage of Environmental Causation of Breast Cancer"; Barbara Adam, Stuart Allan, Cynthia Carter, and Ulrich Beck, eds., *Environmental Risks and the Media* (New York: Routledge, 1999).

117. Ulrich Beck, *Risk Society: Towards a New Modernity* (London: Sage, 1992).

118. Beck, *Risk Society.*

CHAPTER 2   CANCER IN CLYDE AND "WILL-O'-THE-WISP THINGS"

1. Ohio Department of Health (ODH), *Cancer Incidence among Childhood Residents of Clyde City and Green Creek Township, Sandusky County, Ohio, 1996–2006,* Chronic Disease and Behavioral Epidemiology Section and the Ohio Cancer Incidence Surveillance System, Ohio Department of Health and the Sandusky County Department of Public Health, Final Report, April 17, 2007.

2. All cancers diagnosed among Ohio residents on or after January 1, 1992, with the exception of basal and squamous cell carcinoma of the skin and cervical cancer in situ, are required to be reported to OCISS.

3. ODH, *Cancer Incidence among Childhood Residents of Clyde City and Green Creek Township, Sandusky County, Ohio, 1996–2006.*

4. ODH, Sandusky County Health Department, and Ohio Environmental Protection Agency (OEPA), *Childhood Cancer among Residents of Eastern Sandusky County: Progress Report,* October 29, 2009.

5. ODH, Sandusky County Health Department, and OEPA, *Childhood Cancer among Residents of Eastern Sandusky County.*

6. *Fighting for Answers in the Clyde Cancer Cluster,* dir. Adan Garcia (2011).

7. Paul Mohai and Robin Saha, "Which Came First, People or Pollution? Assessing the Disparate Siting and Post-Siting Demographic Change Hypothesis of Environmental Injustice," *Environmental Research Letters* 10, no. 11 (2016): 1–17.

8. Environmental Protection Agency (EPA), "Porcelain Enameling Effluent Guidelines," 2021, https://www.epa.gov/eg/porcelain-enameling-effluent-guidelines.

9. ODH, Sandusky County Health Department, and OEPA, *Childhood Cancer among Residents of Eastern Sandusky County*.

10. EPA, *TRI Facility Report*, accessed July 8, 2018, https://www3.epa.gov/enviro/facts/tri/ef-facilities/#/Chemical/43410WHRLP119BI.

11. OEPA, *Air Quality Report for Clyde and Green Springs*, OEPA Division of Air Pollution Control, May 14, 2010.

12. OEPA, *Water Quality Sampling to Support the Ohio Department of Health Childhood Cancer Investigation, City of Clyde and Surrounding Townships April 9, 2009*, OEPA Division of Drinking and Ground Waters. See also OEPA, *Addendum to Drinking Water Quality Sampling to Support the Ohio Department of Health Childhood Cancer Investigation, City of Clyde and Surrounding Townships*, OEPA Division of Drinking and Ground Waters, August 19, 2009.

13. ODH, *Report on ODH Radiological Screening of 20 Schools in Eastern Sandusky County*, ODH Bureau of Radiation Protection (BRP), Final Report, November 19, 2009.

14. ODH, *Evaluation of Ohio EPA Soil Sampling in Support of the Clyde and Eastern Sandusky County Childhood Cancer Investigation*, ODH Health Assessment Section, July 28, 2011.

15. *19 Action News*, "Ohio's Federal EPA Director Questioned about the Clyde Cancer Cluster," 19actionnews.com, June 17, 2011, accessed May 18, 2014, https://www.cleveland19.com/story/14930336/ohios-epa-director-questioned-about-clyde-cancer-cluster/.

16. Misti Crane, "State Wary of Cancer Clusters but Will Continue Investigations," *Columbus Dispatch*, June 11, 2012, Dispatch.com, accessed May 18, 2014, https://www.dispatch.com/story/lifestyle/health-fitness/2012/06/11/state-wary-cancer-clusters-but/23680220007/.

17. Rev. Edward Pinkey, "Should Whirlpool Pay Taxes?," *People's Tribune*, January 2014, accessed January 5, 2022, http://peoplestribune.org/pt-news/2014/01/whirlpool-pay-taxes/.

18. I reached out to staff at ODH to ask if they assessed the rate of cancer for the adult population for this study, but they were not aware if various types of diseases were assessed in the adult population of Clyde and Green Creek Township during the Clyde childhood cancer investigation.

19. U.S. EPA, *Site Assessment Report Eastern Sandusky County Dumps Site Clyde, Sandusky County, Ohio*, 2012; U.S. EPA—Region 5, Superfund Emergency Response Section, *Site Assessment Report for the Whirlpool Park Site, Green Springs, Sandusky County, Ohio*, July 2012.

20. Weston Solutions, *Site Assessment Report for the Shaw Road Site, Green Springs, Sandusky County, Ohio*, September 27, 2012.

21. U.S. EPA, *Interim Site Assessment Report for the Whirlpool Park Site*, EPA split sampling of the Whirlpool Park site, June 2013.

22. U.S. EPA, *Site Assessment Report for the Whirlpool Park Site, Green Springs, Sandusky County, Ohio*, U.S. EPA—Region 5, Superfund Emergency Response Section, September 2012.

23. Brown v. Whirlpool Corp., 996 F. Supp. 2d 623 (2014).

24. W. M. Kluwe, C. A. Montgomery, H. D. Giles, and J. D. Prejeau, "Encephalopathy in Rats and Nephropathy in Rats and Mice after Subchronic Oral Exposure to Benzaldehyde," *Food and Chemical Toxicology* 21, no. 3 (1983): 245–250.

25. U.S. EPA, "Integrated Risk Information System, Benzaldehyde," 2014, accessed May 21, 2015, http://www.epa.gov/iris/subst/0332.htm.

26. Friedrich Brühne Elaine Wright, "Benzaldehyde," in *Ullmann's Encyclopedia of Industrial Chemistry*, 7th ed. (Hoboken, NJ: Wiley, 2007), 11.

27. ATSDR, Letter to U.S. EPA, ATSDR Region V, June 14, 2013.

28. U.S. EPA, *Interim Site Assessment Report for the Whirlpool Park Site*, U.S. EPA split sampling of the Whirlpool Park site, June 2013.

29. AECOM, *Final Site Assessment Report, Former Whirlpool Park Site, Green Springs, Sandusky County, Ohio*, AECOM, October 29, 2013.

30. U.S. EPA, 2013, Review of Draft Site Assessment Report for the Former Whirlpool Park Site: U.S. EPA letter response to the AECOM Site Assessment Report, October 30, 2013.

31. Tom Jackson, "Report: PCBs Found in Whirlpool Park," *Sandusky Register*, November 1, 2013, SanduskyRegister.com, accessed May 18, 2015.

32. Whirlpool Corporation, *Site Assessment Report Executive Summary, Former Whirlpool Park Site, Green Springs, Sandusky County, Ohio*, October 31, 2013.

33. Tom Henry, "Whirlpool Contractor Exonerates Clyde Site," *Toledo Blade*, November 1, 2013, ToledoBlade.com, May 18, 2014, https://www.toledoblade.com/local/2013/11/01/Whirlpool-contractor-exonerates-Clyde-site/stories/20131031293.

34. Michael J. Thun and Thomas Sinks, "Understanding Cancer Clusters," *CA: A Cancer Journal for Clinicians* 54 (2004): 273–280.

35. Stephen Lester, "Assessing Health Problems in Communities," Center for Health, Environment & Justice, 2010.

36. Adeline Levine, *Love Canal: Science, Politics, and People* (Lexington, MA: Lexington Books, 1982).

37. Strengthening Protections for Children and Communities from Disease Clusters Act, S. 76, 112th Cong. (2011).

38. Stephen Koff, "Senators Want Better Investigations of 'Disease Clusters,' but May Disagree on Methods," Cleveland.com, March 30, 2011, http://www.cleveland.com/open/index.ssf/2011/03/senators_want_better_investiga.html.

39. Thomas E. Shriver and Dennis K. Kennedy, "Contested Environmental Hazards and Community Conflict Over Relocation," *Rural Sociology* 70, no. 4 (2005): 491–513. See also S. M. Capek, "The 'Environmental Justice' Frame: A Conceptual Discussion and an Application," *Social Problems* 40 (1993): 5–24.

40. Ulrich Beck, *Risk Society: Toward a New Modernity* (London: Sage, 1992). See also K. Erikson, "A New Species of Trouble," in *Communities at Risk: Collective Responses to Technological Hazards*, ed. S. R. Couch and J. S. Kroll-Smith (New York: Peter Lang, 1991), 11–29.

41. Thomas E. Shriver and Dennis K. Kennedy, "Contested Environmental Hazards and Community Conflict Over Relocation," *Rural Sociology* 70, no. 4 (2005): 491–513.

42. Javier Auyero and Débora Alejandra Swistun, *Flammable: Environmental Suffering in an Argentine Shantytown* (Oxford: Oxford University Press, 2009), 9.

43. Mary Douglas, *Risk and Blame: Essays in Cultural Theory* (London: Routledge, 1992).

44. Catherine Sanderson, *Why We Act: Turning Bystanders into Moral Rebels* (Cambridge, MA: Harvard University Press, 2020).

45. Philip Mirowski, *Never Let a Serious Crisis Go to Waste* (London: Verso, 2013), 58.

46. Nancy Fraser, "Can Society Be Commodities All the Way Down? Polanyian Reflections on Capitalist Crisis," Fondation Maison des sciences de l'homme, 2012.

47. Sara Ahmed, *The Cultural Politics of Emotion* (Edinburgh, Scotland: Edinburgh University Press, 2004).

CHAPTER 3   EMOTION, RISK, AND OTHERING

1. Doug McAdam and Hilary Boudet, *Putting Social Movements in Their Place: Explaining Opposition to Energy Projects in the United States, 2000–2005* (New York: Cambridge University Press, 2012).

2. Lisa Ritzenhöfer, Prisca Brosi, and Isabell M. Welpe, "Share Your Pride: How Expressing Pride in the Self and Others Heightens the Perception of Agentic and Communal Characteristics," *Journal of Business and Psychology* 34, no. 6 (2019): 847–863.

3. See Felix Septianto, Billy Sung, Yuri Seo, and Nursafwah Tugiman, "Proud Volunteers: The Role of Self- and Vicarious-pride in Promoting Volunteering," *Marketing Letters* 29, no. 4 (December 2018): 501–519; Aaron Ahuvia, Nitika Garg, Rajeev Batra, Brent McFerran, and Pablo Brice Lambert de Diesbach, "Pride of Ownership: An Identity-based Model," *Journal of the Association for Consumer Research* 3, no. 2 (2018): 216–228; Mark H. White II and Nyla R. Branscombe, "'Patriotism à la Carte': Perceived Legitimacy of Collective Guilt and Collective Pride as Motivators for Political Behavior," *Political Psychology* 40, no. 2 (2019): 223–240.; Lisa A. Williams and Joel Davies, "Beyond the Self: Pride Felt in Relation to Others," in *The Moral Psychology of Pride*, ed. J. Adam Carter and Emma C. Gordon (Lanham, MD: Rowman & Littlefield, 2017), 43–68.

4. Michael F. Mascolo and Kurt W. Fischer, "Developmental Transformations in Appraisals for Pride, Shame, and Guilt," in *Self-conscious Emotions: The Psychology of Shame, Guilt, Embarrassment, and Pride*, ed. June Price Tangney and Kurt W. Fischer (New York: Guilford Press, 1995), 64–113.

5. Nicole Syringa Harth, Thomas Kessler, and Colin Wayne Leach, "Advantaged Group's Emotional Reactions to Intergroup Inequality: The Dynamics of Pride, Guilt, and Sympathy," *Personality and Social Psychology Bulletin* 34, no. 1 (2008): 115–129.

6. Alessandro Salice and Alba Montes Sánchez, "Pride, Shame, and Group Identification," *Frontiers in Psychology* 7 (2016): 557.

7. Henrietta Bolló, Beáta Bőthe, István Tóth-Király, and Gábor Orosz, "Pride and Social Status," *Frontiers in Psychology* 9 (October 25, 2018): 1979, doi: 10.3389/fpsyg.2018.01979.

8. Anna Dorfman, Tal Eyal, and Yoella Bereby-Meyer, "Proud to Cooperate: The Consideration of Pride Promotes Cooperation in a Social Dilemma," *Journal of Experimental Social Psychology* 55 (2014): 105–109.

9. Williams and Davies, "Beyond the Self."

10. Erving Goffman, *The Presentation of Self in Everyday Life* (New York: Overlook, 1959).

11. Thomas J. Scheff, "Shame and the Social Bond," *Sociological Theory* 18 (2000): 84–98; Susan Shott, "Emotion and Social Life: A Symbolic Interactionist Analysis," *American Journal of Sociology* 84, no. 6 (1979): 1317–1334.

12. Donald L. Nathanson, ed., *The Many Faces of Shame* (New York: Guilford, 1987).

13. Jessica Fields, Martha Copp, and Sherryl Kleinman, "Symbolic Interactionism, Inequality, and Emotions," in *Handbook of the Sociology of Emotions*, ed. Jonathan H. Turner and Jan E. Stets (Boston: Springer, 2006), 155–178.

14. Scheff, "Shame and the Social Bond."

15. Scheff, "Shame and the Social Bond."

16. BrandsMart USA, "Inside Maytag—American Pride," 2013, accessed December 19, 2020, https://www.youtube.com/watch?v=RSovVO5tS3c.

17. David Roediger, "All about Eve, Critical Whiteness Studies, and Getting over Whiteness," in *Theories of Race and Racism*, ed. Les Back and John Solomos (London: Routledge, 2000), 595–615.

18. David Roediger, *The Wages of Whiteness: Race and the Making of the American Working Class* (London: Verso, 1991).

19. Uma M. Jayakumar and Annie S. Adamian, "The Fifth Frame of Colorblind Ideology: Maintaining the Comforts of Colorblindness in the Context of White Fragility," *Sociological Perspectives* 60, no. 5 (2017): 912–936.

20. Thomas Guglielmo, *White on Arrival: Italians, Race, Color, and Power in Chicago, 1890–1945* (Oxford: Oxford University Press, 2003).

21. Ruth Frankenberg, *The Social Construction of Whiteness: White Women, Race Matters* (Minneapolis: University of Minnesota Press, 1993).

22. Gita Gulati-Pateel and Maggie Potapchuk, "Paying Attention to White Culture and Privilege: A Missing Link to Advancing Racial Equity," *Foundation Review* 6, no. 1 (2014): 25–38.

23. Isabelle Anguelovski, "From Environmental Trauma to Safe Haven: Place Attachment and Place Remaking in Three Marginalized Neighborhoods of Barcelona, Boston, and Havana," *City and Community* 12, no. 3 (2013): 211–237; Melinda J. Milligan, "Displacement and Identity Discontinuity: The Role of Nostalgia in Establishing New Identity Categories," *Symbolic Interaction* 26, no. 3 (2003): 381–403.

24. Pamela Neumann, "Toxic Talk and Collective (In)action in a Company Town: The Case of La Oroya, Peru," *Social Problems* 63, no. 3 (2016): 431–446.

25. Kai Erikson, *A New Species of Trouble: The Human Experience of Modern Disasters* (New York: W. W. Norton, 1994), 111.

26. Thomas F. Gieryn, "A Space for Place in Sociology," *Annual Review of Sociology* 29, no. 1 (2000): 463–496.

27. Andrew Tudor, "A (Macro) Sociology of Fear?," *Sociological Review* 51, no. 2 (2003): 238–256.

28. Joanna Bourke, "Fear and Anxiety: Writing about Emotion in Modern History," *History Workshop Journal* 55 (2003): 111–133.

29. Tudor, "(Macro) Sociology of Fear?," 241.

30. Joanna Bourke, *Fear: A Cultural History* (London: Virago, 2005).

31. Peter Jackson and Jonathan Everts, "Anxiety as Social Practice," *Environment and Planning A* 42, no. 11 (2010): 2791–2806.

32. Mary V. Wrenn, "The Social Ontology of Fear and Neoliberalism," *Review of Social Economy* 72, no. 3 (2014): 337–353.

33. Wrenn, "Social Ontology of Fear and Neoliberalism," 341.

34. Jackson, and Everts, "Anxiety as Social Practice."

35. See Barry Glassner, "The Construction of Fear," *Qualitative Sociology* 22, no. 4 (1999): 301–309.; F. Furedi, *Culture of Fear: Risk-taking and the Morality of Low Expectation* (London: Cassell, 1997).

36. Tudor, "(Macro) Sociology of Fear?," 251.

37. Bourke, *Fear*.

38. Sara Ahmed, *The Cultural Politics of Emotion* (Edinburgh, Scotland: Edinburgh University Press, 2004).

39. Ahmed, *Cultural Politics of Emotion*, 10.

40. Todd L. Matthews, "The Enduring Conflict of 'Jobs versus the Environment': Local Pollution Havens as an Integrative Empirical Measure of Economy versus Environment," *Sociological Spectrum* 31, no. 1 (2010): 59–85; Pamela Neumann, "Toxic Talk and Collective (In)action in a Company Town: The Case of La Oroya, Peru," *Social Problems* 63, no. 3 (2016): 431–446.

41. Shannon Bell, *Fighting King Coal: The Challenges to Micromobilization in Central Appalachia* (Cambridge, MA: MIT Press, 2016); Stephanie A. Malin, *The Price of Nuclear Power: Uranium Communities and Environmental Justice* (New Brunswick, NJ: Rutgers University Press, 2015).

42. Steven Greenhouse, "In Indiana, Centerpiece for a City Closes Shop," *New York Times*, June 19, 2010, https://www.nytimes.com/2010/06/20/us/20whirlpool.html.

43. "Whirlpool Closing Fort Smith Plant," *Arkansas Democratic Gazette*, October 27, 2011, http://www.arkansasonline.com/news/2011/oct/27/whirlpool-closing-fort-smith-plant/.

44. Kari Marie Norgaard, *Living in Denial: Climate Change, Emotions, and Everyday Life* (Cambridge, MA: MIT Press, 2011).

45. Robert J. Lifton, *The Protean Self: Human Resiliency in an Age of Fragmentation* (New York: Basic Books, 1993).

46. Norgaard, *Living in Denial*, 5.

47. Norgaard, *Living in Denial*.

48. Kari Marie Norgaard, "People Want to Protect Themselves a Little Bit: Emotions, Denial, and Social Movement Nonparticipation," *Sociological Inquiry* 76, no. 3 (2006): 372–396.

49. Maricarmen Hernandez, "Building a Home: Everyday Placemaking in a Toxic Neighborhood," *Sociological Perspectives* 62, no. 5 (2019): 709–727.

50. Hernandez, "Building a Home," 711.

51. Ahmed, *Cultural Politics of Emotion*, 17.

52. Eviatar Zerubavel, *Social Mindscapes: An Invitation to Cognitive Sociology* (Cambridge, MA: Harvard University Press, 1997).

53. Zygmunt Bauman, *Modernity and Ambivalence* (Ithaca, NY: Cornell University Press, 1991).

54. Saskia Sassen, *Expulsions: Brutality and Complexity in the Global Economy* (Cambridge, MA: Harvard University Press, 2014).

55. John A. Powell and Stephen Menendian, "The Problem of Othering: Towards Inclusiveness and Belonging," *Othering and Belonging* (Haas Institute for a Fair and Inclusive Society at the University of California, Berkeley) 1 (2018): 14–35; Bauman, *Modernity and Ambivalence*.

56. Powell and Menendian, "Problem of Othering."

57. William R. Freudenburg and Timothy R. Jones, "Attitudes and Stress in the Presence of a Technological Risk: A Test of the Supreme Court Hypothesis," *Social Forces* 69 (1991): 1143–1168.

58. Erikson, *New Species of Trouble*, 236.

59. Erikson, *New Species of Trouble*, 237.

60. See Thomas E. Shriver and Dennis K. Kennedy, "Contested Environmental Hazards and Community Conflict over Relocation," *Rural Sociology* 70, no. 4 (2005): 491–513.

61. William R. Freudenburg and Robert Gramling, *Oil in Troubled Waters: Perceptions, Politics, and the Battle over Offshore Drilling* (Albany: State University of New York Press, 1994).

62. Thomas E. Shriver and Charles Peaden, "Frame Disputes in a Natural Resource Controversy: The Case of the Arbuckle Simpson Aquifer in South-Central Oklahoma," *Society and Natural Resources* 22, no. 2 (2009): 143–157.

63. Alison M. Jagger, "Love and Knowledge: Emotion in Feminist Epistemology," in *Gender/Body/Knowledge: Feminist Reconstructions of Being and Knowing*, ed. Alison M. Jagger and Susan Bordo (New Brunswick, NJ: Rutgers University Press, 1989).

64. Arthur Kleinman, "Experience and Its Moral Modes: Culture, Human Conditions, and Disorder: The Tanner Lectures on Human Values" (Presented at Stanford University, April 13–16, Palo Alto, CA, 1998), 365.

65. Thomas Osborne, "Of Health and Statecraft," in *Foucault, Health and Medicine*, ed. Robin Bunton and Alan Petersen (New York: Routledge, 1997), 173–188.

66. Ahmed, *Cultural Politics of Emotion*, 3–4, 10.

67. Pamela Neumann, "Toxic Talk and Collective (In)action in a Company Town: The Case of La Oroya, Peru," *Social Problems* 63, no. 3 (2016): 431–446.

68. The year 2018 is the most current and complete year of cancer incidence data available from the Ohio Cancer Incidence Surveillance System (OCISS). Based on OCISS geocoded data, a total of eight malignant cancer cases were diagnosed from 2011 to 2018 (among children and adolescents aged 0–19) of Clyde City and Green Creek Township. Five cases resided within Clyde City Limits, and three cases resided in the remainder of Green Creek Township.

69. See Erikson, *New Species of Trouble*.

CHAPTER 4   EMBODIED RISK

1. Anne M. Kavanagh and Dorothy H. Broom, "Embodied Risk: My Body, Myself?," *Social Science & Medicine* 46, no. 3 (1998): 442.

2. Kavanagh and Broom, "Embodied Risk," 442.

3. Gustaf Ljungman, T. Gordh, S. Sorensen, and A. Kreuger, "Pain Variations during Cancer Treatment in Children: A Descriptive Survey," *Pediatric Hematology and Oncology* 17 (2000): 211–221.

4. Gregory Weiss and Lynne E. Lonnquist, *The Sociology of Health, Healing, and Illness*, 9th ed. (New York: Routledge, 2017).

5. Imelda Oktaviani and Allenidekania Allenidekania, "Correlation between Parents' Self-efficacy and Quality of Life of Children with Cancer Aged 8–12 Years," *Pediatric Reports* 12, no. 1 (2020): 52–56; Lynnda M. Dahlquist, Danita I. Czyzewski, and Cheri L. Jones, "Parents of Children with Cancer: A Longitudinal Study of Emotional Distress, Coping Style, and Marital Adjustment Two and Twenty Months after Diagnosis," *Journal of Pediatric Psychology* 21, no. 4 (1995): 541–554.

6. L. M. Massimo, T. J. Wiley, and E. F. Casari, "From Informed Consent to Shared Consent: A Developing Process in Pediatric Oncology," *Lancet Oncology* 5 (2004): 384–387; G. Ljungman, T. Gordh, S. Sörensen, and A. Kreuger, "Pain in Pediatric Oncology: Interviews with Children, Adolescents and their Parents," *Acta Pædiatrica* 88 (1999): 623–630.

7. Kelly James, Diane Keegan-Wells, Pamela S. Hinds, Katherine P. Kelly, Dana Bond, Brenda Hall, Rosemary Mahan, Ida M. Moore, Lona Roll, and Beth Speckhart, "The Care of My Child with Cancer: Parents' Perceptions of Caregiving Demands," *Journal of Pediatric Oncology Nursing* 19, no. 6 (2002): 218–228.

8. William J. Goode, "A Theory of Role Strain," *American Sociological Review* 25, no. 4 (1960): 483–496; J.R.P. French and R. D. Caplan, "Organizational Stress and Individual Strain," in *The Failure of Success*, ed. Alfred J. Morrow (New York: Amacom, 1973), 30–66.

9. Akhtar Iqbal and Khawer S. Siddiqui, "Depression among Parents of Children with Acute Lymphoblastic Leukemia," *Joournal of Ayub Medical College Abbottabad* 14, no. 2 (2002): 6–9; L. von Essen, P. O. Sjoden, and E. Mattsson, "Swedish Mothers and Fathers of a Child Diagnosed with Cancer: A Look at Their Quality of Life," *Acta Oncologica* 43, no. 5 (2004): 474–479; C. H. Yeh, "Gender Differences of Parental Distress in Children with Cancer," *Journal of Advanced Nursing* 38, no. 6 (2002): 598–606; Melissa A. Alderfer, Avital Cnaan, Rachel A. Annunziato, and Anne E. Kazak, "Patterns of Posttraumatic Stress Symptoms in Parents of Childhood Cancer Survivors," *Journal of Family Psychology* 19, no. 3 (2005): 430–440.

10. Viktor Gecas and Peter J. Burke, "Self and Identity," in *Sociological Perspectives on Social Psychology* (New York: Basic Books, 1995), 41–67.

11. Oscar A. Barbarin, Diane Hughes, and Mark A. Chesler, "Stress, Coping and Marital Function among Parents of Children with Cancer," *Applied Psychology* 47, no. 2 (1985): 473–480.

12. Barbarin, Hughes, and Chesler, "Stress, Coping and Marital Function."

13. Adi Ophir, "The Politics of Catastrophization: Emergency and Exception," in *Contemporary States of Emergency: The Politics of Military and Humanitarian Interventions*, ed. Didier Fassin and Mariella Pandolfi (New York: Zone Books, 2010), 40–61.

14. Mark Novak and Carol Guest, "Application of a Multidimensional Caregiver Burden Inventory," *Gerontologist* 29, no. 6 (1989): 798–803.

15. Novak and Guest, "Application."

16. Jacques Derrida, *Given Time: I. Counterfeit Money* (Chicago: University of Chicago Press, 1994).

17. Kai Erikson, *A New Species of Trouble: The Human Experience of Modern Disasters* (New York: W. W. Norton, 1994).

18. Michael R. Edelstein, *Contaminated Communities: Coping with Residential Toxic Exposure* (Boulder, CO: Westview, 2004).

19. Michael Edelstein, "Toxic Exposure and the Inversion of the Home," *Journal of Architectural and Planning Research* 3, no. 3 (1986): 237–251.

20. Dayna Scott, "Risk as a Technique of Governance in an Era of Biotechnological Innovation: Implications for Democratic Citizenship and Strategies of Resistance," in *Risk and Trust: Including or Excluding Citizens?*, ed. Law Commission of Canada (Black Point, N.S.: Fernwood, 2007), 23–56.

21. Norah McKendrick, *Better Safe than Sorry: How Consumers Navigate Exposure to Everyday Toxics* (Oakland: University of California Press, 2018).

22. See Michael Maniates, "Individualization: Plant a Tree, Buy a Bike, Save the World?," *Global Environmental Politics* 1, no. 3 (2001): 31–52.

CHAPTER 5   TOWARD TRANSFORMATIVE MOVEMENTS OF THEORY AND PRACTICE

1. In the mid-1990s, the Ohio EPA began receiving complaints from Wellington residents regarding dust fallout and odors from the Sterling Foundry, a facility that produced gray and ductile iron castings, primarily for heavy industry. Shortly after these complaints were made, Wellington residents began to voice concerns about environmental toxins and the high rates of illness within their community. A 1998 study by the Ohio Department of Health and the Lorain County Health Department, which used data from the National Health Interview Survey, identified that residents there were 3.7 times more likely to develop multiple sclerosis (MS) than the rest of the country. Wellington residents also expressed concerns about the occurrences of cancer, fibromyalgia, and lupus within their community. In 2003, a resident petitioned the Agency for Toxic Substances and Disease Registry (ATSDR) to conduct a public health assessment. Although environmental contaminants and local industries were implicated, experts were unable to pinpoint the exact cause of the higher rates of disease within the community. No additional sampling was recommended by ATSDR, in part because of the closing of the local facilities in question.

In the late 1990s in Marion County, Ohio, residents began questioning the high cancer rates among graduates of the River Valley schools. The Ohio EPA discovered that the high school and middle school were built on a former U.S. Army waste dump where students could have been exposed to more than seventy-five hazardous contaminants. After families fought to close the schools, the district relocated the schools three miles away. However, the state health department ended the investigation of eighty-three leukemia cases after five years without determining a cause because of a lack of direct evidence that the chemicals caused the cancer. Marysville, Ohio, is the location of another leukemia cluster, the cause of which also remains unknown.

2. Somerville, Texas, a town of approximately 1,400 people, about 60 percent of whom are Black or Hispanic, is home to a large wood-treatment facility that locals call the "tie plant," once the nation's largest producer of railroad cross-ties. In the late 1990s, its residents began noticing high rates of birth defects and cancers of the brain and stomach within the community. Environmental scientists identified extremely high levels of cancer-causing chemicals in the dust of Somerville homes and school buildings. As reported by a comprehensive Houston Press investigation, residents were contracting stomach cancer at a rate as much as forty to sixty times the national average. In response to residents' concerns, the Texas Department of

Public Health Services conducted epidemiological studies but did not find that the incidence of cancer was significantly different from the national average. Some impacted residents sued the local company, alleging that the company sprayed toxic pesticides throughout the facility, burned creosote-treated wood in boiler stacks at night to avoid complaints from townspeople, destroyed company documents, and failed to provide employees with proper safety equipment. Creosote, which the International Agency for Research on Cancer and the EPA have determined is likely a carcinogen, is a large mixture of chemicals that is used in the United States as a wood preservative, as well as for roofing, aluminum smelting, and road paving. The tie plant even "provided families with metal barrels that once contained pesticides to use as makeshift barbecues." Several employees recounted receiving instructions from company managers to conduct these harmful practices, noting that their jobs depended on fulfilling these requests. Yet former managers and city officials downplayed the cancer problem in Somerville and placed responsibility for protection from industrial contaminants on the plant workers. In response to the class-action lawsuit, one company spokesman stated, "It is our position that there is no reliable scientific evidence to support their claims."

Like Clyde, Flint is located in what is considered the Rust Belt and was once the location of the largest General Motors plant. Flint began to decline in the 1980s when GM downsized. In this case, re-sourcing of the city's water supply was initiated as a cost-saving measure, and the city's water source was diverted from Lake Huron to the heavily polluted Flint River. This move ultimately corroded the city's older pipe delivery system and leached lead into the sinks and showers of a city of approximately 100,000 people, with children emerging as the most vulnerable victims of the contamination.

Public officials were instrumental in changing the water system to save money that negatively affected water quality. Flint's mayor, U.S. EPA officials, and emergency managers repeatedly told concerned residents that the water was fine and were slow to correct the problem. Finally, a lead water pipe removal program was established in 2017 because of a court order in response to a lawsuit by Flint residents. By September 2021, the city had replaced more than 10,000 lead pipes, although lead remains inside older homes, in plumbing fixtures and galvanized pipes, and many Flint residents continue to worry about their drinking water and do not trust that the lead problem has been remedied.

Systems of power operating across communities impacted by industrial contamination are similar. In contrast to Clyde, though, the source of toxicity was definitively identified in Flint. Compared with Clyde, the problem in Flint has impacted the whole community, was more immediately recognized as a crisis, has received enormous public attention, and awakened perceptions of the presence of lead in the water of other communities, and yet residents remain distrustful.

3. Courtney Cuthbertson, Cathy Newkirk, Joan Ilardo, Scott Loveridge, and Mark Skidmore, "Angry, Scared, and Unsure: Mental Health Consequences of Contaminated Water in Flint, Michigan," *Journal of Urban Health* 93, no. 6 (December 2016): 899–908. In their study of Black and White residents living in or around the environmentally contaminated Red River community of Clarksville, Tennessee, Robert Emmet Jones and Shirley A. Rainey found that Blacks are more likely than Whites to believe they are being exposed to poorer environmental conditions, suffer more health-related problems, and think that local public agencies and officials have not dealt with environmental problems in their neighborhood in a just, equitable, and effective manner. See Robert Emmet Jones and Shirley A. Rainey, "Examining Linkages between Race, Environmental Concern, Health, and Justice in a Highly Polluted Community of Color," *Journal of Black Studies* 36, no. 4 (2006): 473–496.

4. Celene Krause, "Women of Color on the Frontline," in *Unequal Protection: Environmental Justice and Communities of Color*, ed. Robert D. Bullard (San Francisco, CA: Sierra Club, 1994), 256–271.

5. See Robert Bullard, *Dumping in Dixie: Race, Class, and Environmental Quality* (Boulder, CO: Westview, 2000).

6. Bullard, *Dumping in Dixie*.

7. Robert Higgens, "Race, Pollution and the Mastery of Nature," *Environmental Ethics* 16 (1994): 251–263.

8. Robin S. Gregory and Theresa A Satterfield, "Beyond Perception: The Experience of Risk and Stigma in Community Contexts," *Risk Analysis* 22, no. 2 (April 2002): 347–358.

9. Rebecca S. Bigler and Caitlin Clark, "The Inherence Heuristic: A Key Theoretical Addition to Understanding Social Stereotyping and Prejudice," *Behavioral and Brain Sciences* 37, no. 5 (2014): 483–484.

10. Emily Huddart Kennedy and Josée Johnston, "If You Love the Environment, Why Don't You Do Something to Save It? Bringing Culture into Environmental Analysis," *Sociological Perspectives* 62, no. 5 (2019): 593–602.

11. Rebecca Lave, Philip Mirowski, and Samuel Randalls, "Introduction: STS and Neoliberal Science," *Social Studies of Science* 40, no. 5 (2010): 659–675.

12. Kelly Moore, Daniel Lee Kleinman, David Hess, and Scott Frickel, "Science and Neoliberal Globalization: A Political Sociological Approach," *Theory and Society* 40 (2001): 505–532.

13. Public opinion about science is as complex as the scientific enterprise itself, and generally, some public divisions over science, such as those related to climate and energy issues, are aligned with partisanship, while others are not. Partisan differences in overall views and trust in scientists is especially pronounced for environmental scientists. See Pew Research Center, "Trust and Mistrust in Americans' Views of Scientific Experts," 2019, https://www.pewresearch .org/science/2019/08/02/trust-and-mistrust-in-americans-views-of-scientific-experts/.

14. Exec. Order No. 13783, FR 31396 (March 28, 2017).

15. United States, 115th Congress, Pub. L. No. 115–5, *H.J. Res. 38, Joint Resolution: Disapproving the rule submitted by the Department of the Interior known as the Stream Protection Rule* (Washington, DC: U.S. G.P.O., 2017).

16. U.S. Environmental Protection Agency, *Notice Regarding Withdrawal of Obligation to Submit Information*, 82 FR 12817 (Washington, DC, 2017).

17. U.S. Environmental Protection Agency, Office of Chemical Safety and Pollution Prevention, *Chlorpyrifos: Revised Human Health Risk Assessment for Registration Review* (Washington, DC, 2016); U.S. Environmental Protection Agency, *Chlorpyrifos; Order Denying PANNA and NRDC's Petition to Revoke Tolerances*, 82 FR 16581 (Washington, DC, 2017); Virginia A. Rauh, Frederica P. Perera, Megan K. Horton, Robin M. Whyatt, Ravi Bansal, Xuejun Hao, Jun Liu, Dana Boyd Barr, Theodore A. Slotkin, and Bradley S. Peterson, "Brain Anomalies in Children Exposed Prenatally to a Common Organophosphate Pesticide," *Proceedings of the National Academy of Sciences* 109, no. 20 (April 30, 2012): 7871–7876.

18. Eric Lipton, "The Chemical Industry Scores a Big Win at the E.P.A.," *New York Times*, June 7, 2018, A1.

19. PFAS for decades have been used to make thousands of products water- and stain-resistant such as fire retardants, furniture, and nonstick cookware. When lawmakers introduced over a hundred new pieces of legislation aimed at regulating PFAS in 2019 and 2020, industry spending on PFAS issues increased. Chemours, a top PFAS manufacturer, reported $5 billion in earnings in 2020, about one-quarter of which came from fluorinated chemicals.

20. U.S. Department of the Interior, "Climate Change," accessed July 24, 2018, https://web .archive.org/web/20170225220625/https://www.doi.gov/climate.

21. Coral Davenport, "How Much Has 'Climate Change' Been Scrubbed from Federal Websites? A Lot," *New York Times*, January 10, 2018, https://www.nytimes.com/2018/01/10/climate /climate-change-trump.html.

22. Warren Cornwall, "New Rule Could Force EPA to Ignore Major Human Health Studies," *Science*, April 25, 2018, accessed October 12, 2018, https://www.sciencemag.org/news/2018/04/new-rule-could-force-epa-ignore-major-human-health-studies.

23. Environmental Integrity Project, "Civil Penalties against Polluters Drop 60 Percent So Far under Trump," August 10, 2017, http://www.environmentalintegrity.org/news/penalties-drop-under-trump/.

24. U.S. Department of the Interior, Office of Surface Mining Reclamation and Enforcement, letter from Acting Director Glenda H. Owens to Elizabeth A. Eide, senior board director, Board on Earth Sciences and Resources, Water and Technology Board, National Academies of Sciences, Engineering, and Medicine, August 18, 2017, https://www.documentcloud.org/documents/3936617-Interior-Stop-Work-Letter-to-NAS.html; Paul Voosen, "NASA Cancels Carbon Monitoring Research Program," *Science* 360, no. 6389 (May 11, 2018): 586–587.

25. Tom Perkins, "How US Chemical Industry Lobbying and Cash Defeated Regulation in Trump Era," *Guardian*, April 26, 2021, https://www.theguardian.com/environment/2021/apr/26/us-chemical-companies-lobbying-donation-defeated-regulation.

26. Jon P. Devine, "Has There Been a Corporate Takeover of EPA Science?," *Risk Policy Report* 8 (2001): 35–38.

27. Tuukka Ylä-Anttila, "Populist Knowledge: 'Post-truth' Repertoires of Contesting Epistemic Authorities," *European Journal of Cultural and Political Sociology* 5, no. 4 (2018): 356–388.

28. Lorenzo Mosca and Donatella della Porta, "Unconventional Politics Online: Internet and the Global Justice Movement," in *Democracy in Social Movements*, ed. Donatella della Porta (Basingstoke: Palgrave Macmillan, 2009), 194–216.

29. Cary Funk, "Key Findings about Americans' Confidence in Science and Their Views on Scientists' Role in Society," Pew Research Center, February 12, 2020, https://www.pewresearch.org/fact-tank/2020/02/12/key-findings-about-americans-confidence-in-science-and-their-views-on-scientists-role-in-society/.

30. Clara Voyvodic Casabó, "Post-Truth Politics and the Fracture of Neo-liberalism's 'Double-truth' Doctrine: Governmentality and Resistance in the US and the UK," *St. Antony's International Review* 13, no. 2 (2018): 48–63.

31. Jürgen Habermas, *Theory of Communicative Action*, trans. Thomas McCarthy (Boston: Beacon, 1987).

32. Habermas, *Theory of Communicative Action*.

33. Feeding America, "The Impact of the Coronavirus on Food Insecurity in 2020 & 2021," 2021, accessed January 3, 2022, https://www.feedingamerica.org/sites/default/files/2021-03/National%20Projections%20Brief_3.9.2021_0.pdf.

34. Rong Wang, Liu Hongyun, Jiang Jiang, and Yue Song, "Will Materialism Lead to Happiness? A Longitudinal Analysis of the Mediating Role of Psychological Needs Satisfaction," *Personality and Individual Differences* 105 (2017): 312–317; Jose A. Muñiz-Velázquez, Diego Gomez-Baya, and Manuel Lopez-Casquete, "Implicit and Explicit Assessment of Materialism: Associations with Happiness and Depression," *Personality and Individual Differences* 116 (2017): 123–132; Jonathan E. Schroeder and Sanjiv S. Dugal, "Psychological Correlates of the Materialism Construct," *Journal of Social Behavior and Personality* 10, no. 1 (1995): 243.

35. Tim Kasser, Richard M. Ryan, Charles E. Couchman, and Kennon M. Sheldon, "Materialistic Values: Their Causes and Consequences," in *Psychology and Consumer Culture: The Struggle for a Good Life in a Materialistic World*, ed. Tim Kasser and Allen D. Kanner (Washington, DC: American Psychological Association, 2004), 11–28.

36. Thomas Scheff, "Goffman on Emotions: The Pride-Shame System," *Symbolic Interaction* 37, no. 1 (2013): 108–121.

37. Sara Ahmed, *The Cultural Politics of Emotion* (Edinburgh, Scotland: Edinburgh University Press, 2004), 11.

38. Stephen Gill, "New Constitutionalism, Democratisation and Global Political Economy," *Pacifica Review* 10, no. 1 (1998): 23–38.

39. Amanda Lewis, "What Group?: Studying Whites and Whiteness in the Era of Color-blindness," *Sociological Theory* 22, no. 4 (2004): 623–646.

40. Emily Feng, "Why the Chinese Government Wants More Feel-Good Stories Posted Online," *Morning Edition* on NPR, January 10, 2022, https://www.npr.org/2022/01/10/1071766938/why-the-chinese-government-wants-more-feel-good-stories-posted-online.

41. John R. Hibbing and Elizabeth Theiss-Morse, *Stealth Democracy: Americans' Beliefs about How Government Should Work* (New York: Cambridge University Press, 2002).

42. Lois Gibbs, Public Meeting on Fracking & Injection Well Concerns, Youngstown, Ohio, March 13, 2015.

43. Nikolay L. Mihaylov and Douglas D. Perkins, "Local Environmental Grassroots Activism: Contributions from Environmental Psychology, Sociology and Politics," *Behavioral Sciences* 5, no. 1 (2015): 121–153.

44. Dayna Nadine Scott, "Shifting the Burden of Proof: the Precautionary Principle and Its Potential for the 'Democratization' of Risk," in *Law and Risk*, ed. Law Commission of Canada (Vancouver: UBC Press and Les Presses de L'Université Laval, 2005), 50–85.

45. Jeanne M. Stellman, Steven D. Stellman, Richard Christian, Tracy Weber, and Carrie Tomasallo, "The Extent and Patterns of Usage of Agent Orange and Other Herbicides in Vietnam," *Nature* 17 (2003): 681–687; Steven D. Stellman and Jeanne M. Stellman, "Exposure Opportunity Models for Agent Orange, Dioxin, and Other Military Herbicides Used in Vietnam, 1961–1971," *Journal of Exposure Analysis and Environmental Epidemiology* 14 (2004): 354–362.

46. Center for Health and Environmental Justice, *Protecting People Exposed to Toxic Chemicals: A New Approach* (Falls Church, VA: Center for Health and Environmental Justice, 2022).

47. California Office of Environmental Health Hazard Assessment, Proposition 65, Safe Drinking Water and Toxic Enforcement Act of 1986, accessed January 4, 2022, https://oehha.ca.gov/proposition-65.

48. Margrit Shildrick, *Leaky Bodies and Boundaries: Feminism, Postmodernism and (Bio)ethics* (London: Routledge, 1997); Stacy Alaimo, "Trans-corporeal Feminisms and the Ethical Space of Nature," in *Material Feminisms*, ed. Stacy Alaimo and Susan Hekman (Bloomington: Indiana University Press, 2008), 237–264.

49. Dayna Scott, Jennie Haw, and Robyn Lee, "'Wannabe Toxic-Free?' From Precautionary Consumption to Corporeal Citizenship," *Environmental Politics* 25, no. 6 (2016): 1–21.

50. Émile Durkheim, *The Division of Labor in Society*, trans. George Simpson (New York: Free Press of Glencoe, 1964).

51. Kirstin Dow, Frans Berkhout, and Benjamin L. Preston, "Limits to Adaptation to Climate Change: A Risk Approach," *Current Opinion in Environmental Sustainability* 5, no. 3–4 (2013): 384–391.

INDEX

Pages in italics refer to illustrative matter.

ABOUT THE AUTHOR

LAURA HART is an assistant professor of sociology at Missouri State University in the areas of health and environment.

Printed and bound by CPI Group (UK) Ltd, Croydon, CR0 4YY

27/10/2024

14580231-0005